1001 Easy Powerful Ways to Beat Infertility and Have The Babies You Deserve!

Other Books by the Author:

Dancing Your Way to Fertility
The Infertility Diaries
The Turning 50 Portrait
Early Morning Coffee: Laugh Out Loud Stories about My Life as a Mom
Tree House Cupcake Girls
Your Perfect Wedding
Diary in the Bed
Izzy and the Ice Skating Bakery
Stop Bullying Forever
Tonight at the Fire pit
The Hope Chest
Its Not Your Fault Adam
Cat Tales: My Family and The Cats We Have Loved
Ask The Love Lady
Transference
Sarah and The Sunrock
Sunday at Grandma's
Sunday With Uncle Charlie
Tonight at Salisbury Beach

Visit www.paulafuocodavis.com to learn more!

Paula Fuoco Davis
PaulaMediaandEntertainment.com, Nashua, NH
ISBN:
Edition Notice
Date of Publication: December 30, 2016
Number of Printings: First printing
Year of publication: 2016

Books may be purchased by contacting the publisher and author at dancingyourwaytofertility.com

Books may be purchased in quantity and/or special sales by contacting the publisher, PaulaMediaandEntertainment.com or by email at books@paulamediaandentertainment.com.

Library of Congress Catalog Number:

ISBN:
1. Infertility 2. Fertility 3. Health

First Edition

This book is dedicated to my mother, Sarah Fuoco for being the best mother in the world. You embody what motherhood is in every way. I have always loved and will always love sitting across from you at the kitchen table talking. There is no place I rather be.

My father, Joseph Fuoco, for taking such good care of me and Mom, and working so hard and responsibly to make life beautiful for us. You were a fun Dad, smart, generous and loving. How can I even begin to thank you for all you have given me? You are a beautiful person.

My beautiful children, Amber and Sammy, who God sent as an answer to all my prayers. You were worth every part of this journey, every needle, every minute..all so worth it because having you both has been the most wonderful part of my life. You both fill my days with more joy than you can imagine.

Most of all, I dedicate this book to Jehovah God, the one who answers all prayers and without prayer, I don't know what I would have done.

My best friend, Leah Page Mortimer, who walked with me and helped me every step of the way. You were there during my darkest times, offering hope, acceptance, love, understanding. Yes, you are a genius! And for all the times you said exactly what I needed to hear, thank you.

My husband, Christopher Davis, for being there and walking this hard road with me. You were brave and kind, a true hero, and without you, I would not have my kids. There is no one else I would have rather walked this road with. You helped me give birth to these beautiful children and I can't thank you enough.

1001 Ways

1. When things get rough, remember that infertility may be the best training ground for motherhood ever. This road, this test, this initiation, will test all of you--and it will make you one of the strongest, most capable, confident, resourceful, perseverant mothers a child could ever have. Experiencing infertility gives you a lifetime pass to enjoy motherhood in a way few ever get to enjoy it, because with the difficulties of this disease come confidence and appreciation. This journey will demand all the best parts of you. It will demand you persevere when you want to give up. It will demand patience and persistence when frustration and helpless surrender might feel like a more natural path. It will demand that every survival skill you possess be brought forth and utilized. It will demand sacrifice, self-preservation, and a willpower beyond what you knew you had, but what intrinsically you knew you were capable of.

You have probably been through the best training course for motherhood possible: you understand pain, you understand the potential for joy, you are willing to do the work to get the child you want, and you've proven you can take the bad stuff that comes with going after the good stuff. In doing this, you will join a group of super cultivated mothers, women ready to nurture and love the next generation, and have more than proven their worth to do this.It is an initiation rite, of sorts, an involuntary one, of course. No one should have to go through this to have a baby and no one would voluntarily choose this road. Nonetheless, it is a reality for many of us, and it will prepare you for motherhood in a grand and inspiring way that someday you may even feel thankful to have experienced.

It isn't fair but you still can end up with what everybody else has. It is a long road and an unfair one, but at the end of the road, you could be holding the baby of your dreams, just as the same as someone who made love one night and woke up pregnant the next morning.

Then nothing at all will matter but your baby.

2. You are going to hear no. Expect to hear it at times, but don't let hearing it keep you down or stop you from going after your dream.

3. You are going to have to put some aspects of your life on hold. It will be worth it, but be prepared to spend your time, energy and money on getting pregnant and putting certain aspects of your life on hold.

4. You are going to hear negative comments, sometimes even from the people you love. Don't pay attention to what they say. This can work out for you, despite what anyone says or thinks about your health or situation.

5. This is a journey you might sometimes take alone. Don't be surprised if sometimes even your husband can't be there for you the way you need him to. If that happens, don't waste your time getting angry--just keep going.

6. The doctor you choose and the reproductive clinic they are associated with matters—choose a good one. You want a doctor who is open to trying new medications and procedures and who answers your questions and listens to what you have to say.

7. You are going to have to eat and take care of your body in a way you never have before. Get ready to make spinach, garlic and pumpkin seeds your new best friends.

8. You are going to have to be strong and stay positive, even when nothing positive is happening. You are going to have to get ready to harness every little bit of inner strength you've ever had.

9. You are also going to fall apart sometimes. Just expect it.

10. It is going to feel rotten to be invited to baby showers, children's parties, and see pregnant women at the supermarket. When that happens, just remember: someday, it could very well be you having that baby shower, hosting the children's parties and being that beautiful pregnant lady at the supermarket. And you never know: that mother with the beautiful baby that made your heart ache? She might have once been a fertility patient too.

11. You are going to have to work hard and be flexible. It is important to understand that a lot of work may be required to beat infertility. Infertility treatments require going to lots of appointments, and doing whatever you can to improve your health. This journey takes effort and push. Accepting the hard work involved will make it easier, and hopefully empower you to do what is available to heal your infertility. While beating infertility can be really hard work, the reward it well worth any effort you have to make.

12. Remember: Infertility is not a final statement on your ability to have the family you dream of—infertility is a medical condition that, with the right treatments, is often temporary and can be cured. So starting today, see your infertility as a temporary condition that is a signal that your body is off-track and needs something to heal it.

13. The first step to overcoming infertility is to change the track your body is on from:

• A state of disease and dysfunction to one of health

• An acidic state to an alkaline state

• A state of clogged toxins in the body, to one of a cleansed body with all your organs cleansed and able to function at their highest level possible.

What can set the body down a wrong course? Unhealthy foods, low-quality drinking water, chemicals or toxins in our environment and in products we use, stress, traumas and painful life experiences that tire and weaken our organs.

14. Buy a juicer or a fruit/vegetable drink mixer. Learn as much as you can about making healthy vegetable and fruit drinks. Make this a daily part of your routine, whether it is simply juicing a bag of spinach or making a spinach/blueberry/flaxseed drink.

15. Find a reputable, licensed acupuncturist in your area and start going once, twice or even three times a week.

16. Visit a local health or nature food store and purchase a liver cleanse. You may want to do this more than once. This is to be done before you are in the midst of an IUI or IVF cycle.

17. Visit a supermarket and stock up on garlic, spinach, pumpkin seeds, sunflower seeds, kale, yams, and pineapple.

18. Schedule 20 minutes in your day to sit outside in the sunshine. Pick a place that feels comfortable—even if it is just putting a chair out in your front yard, a driveway or at a local park.

19. Find an excellent, highly reputable chiropractor in your area who is somewhat familiar with issues of infertility who can adjust your spine.

20. Start eating as much spinach and garlic as you can.

21. Get more sleep. Make sure your room is completely dark and get to bed earlier.

22. Stop drinking coffee and eating sugar.

23. Stop all trans fats that are in your diet. Cut down on white flour products too.

24. As always check with a physician before pursuing any course of treatment.

25. Go to your primary care physician and request a complete work-up.

You need to find out if you have:

• Gallstones

• Blood problems or disorders, such as anemia

26. Ask for a complete work-up of your thyroid, liver and kidneys. This includes a thyroid stimulating hormone test and a comprehensive metabolic panel.

27. Get tested for allergies, as you could be eating a food that weakens your body, such as gluten.

28. Have your white blood cell count checked. This might help in determining if there is an undetected infection in your body.

The aim of the physical is to find out if there is an area in your body that has been overlooked, because one weak area can throw off the rest of the body.

29. Visit Your Dentist: Get a complete dental check-up to be sure there are no lingering or untreated infections in your mouth.

30. **Do A Liver Cleanse:** The liver is a highly influential organ that plays a key role in fertility and is one of the most important organs in your body. The liver governs approximately 500 metabolic processes and many studies have shown that the oestrogen receptors in the liver are critical for maintaining fertility.

In addition to a liver cleanse, here are some other ways to detoxify, cleanse and strengthen your liver:

31. Milk thistle is a wonderful herb for cleansing the liver. Read the directions on the bottle carefully as to amounts taken.

32. Lemon is a great liver cleanser. About 20 minutes before breakfast in the morning, squeeze the juice from one or two fresh lemons into some warm water and drink.

33. Beets are excellent liver cleansers. You can eat them cooked or juice them. To juice beets, peel and cut into small wedges that can easily fit in your juicer. Juice the beets with some apple, spinach or kale.

34. Chlorophyll is a highly esteemed liver cleanser.

35. Artichokes are powerful liver protectors because they contain a flavonoid called silymarin, which is an antioxidant that protects the liver from toxicity.

36. Foods that are good for your liver include: spirulina, garlic, carrots, romaine lettuce, apples, grapefruit, chicory, mustard greens, dandelion greens, avocados, walnuts, turmeric and parsley.

37. Cabbage can also be juiced and is effective in cleaning the liver.

38. Amino acids, derived from healthy sources of protein, are key to the liver working at maximum capacity. Foods that contain these amino acids include: nuts, such as pumpkin seeds, squash seeds and almonds; lean meats, eggs, and beans, such as lentils and garbanzo.

39. In Chinese medicine, infertility is often linked to Liver chi stagnation, a result of stress, overwork, and the effects of coffee and alcohol. Irritability, headaches and frustration are just some of the physical and emotional symptoms of liver chi stagnation. Acupuncturists and herbalists can work on unblocking energy stagnation in the liver.

40. According to Chinese medicine, emotional and lifestyle cures for liver stagnation include being assertive, making clear decisions and enjoying lots of fun, laughter and relaxation. Holding on to anger, feeling stuck and depression impair the liver by stagnating the energy. Letting go, moving on, and exercising control over one's life, can help in healing the liver.

41. **Heavy Metal Cleanse:** Every day, we come into contact with heavy metals that can disrupt our fertility. As much as possible, you'll want to start paying attention to the metals you may be unintentionally bringing into your body through the products you use and your lifestyles choices.

Because heavy metals are so common in our world, most of us have them in our systems.

There are a variety of heavy metal cleanses available online and in health food stores. You may want to do this cleanse more than once. This is, however, a cleanse to be done before you start infertility treatments and medications.

Along with a heavy metal cleanse, here are some additional ways to cleanse your body of heavy metals:

42. Avoid Cosmetics, drinking soda straight from a can, deodorants that contain aluminum, solvents in dry cleaning, exposure to radiation, all contain metals that can find their way into our body, causing metabolic disruptions in organs, such as our heart, brain, kidneys and liver.

43. Garlic is known to help reduce metal levels in the body. It contains the antioxidant allicin. You can eat garlic raw, cook with it or juice it.

44. Milk thistle is an herb that can also help remove heavy metals from the liver.

45. Cilantro is a powerful herb that is known for binding heavy metals and whisking them out of the body.

46. Alpha Lipoic Acid and Gluthatione are powerful supplements for helping cells remove heavy metals from the body.

47. Chlorella is a fresh water algae loaded with chlorophyll. Buy it in powder form and mix with water for fast absorption. It can also be taken in capsule or tablet form.

48. A steam bath can help remove metals.

49. Burdock is a potent blood purifier and can remove heavy metals from the body. It also helps purify the liver.

50. Onions contain the antioxidant quercetin, which helps remove heavy metals from the body. Add to your salads daily or juice them.

51. **A Yeast Cleanse:** Yeast, also known as candida, can impact your fertility by causing your internal vagina's flora to become unbalanced, making it difficult for sperm to reach the uterus. Getting rid of yeast is an important step in rebalancing your body so it can heal itself.

Some additional ways to rid your body of yeast:

52. Do a yeast or candida cleanse, that can be bought online, at health food store or nature food store. Acidophillus can help control candida.

53. Flaxseed is known to help control yeast.

54. Garlic is an enemy of yeast. Take garlic capsules, juice garlic and eat lots of raw garlic.

55. Avoid sugar and white flour foods. These can include sugary juices, desserts, breads, crackers, pre-packaged meals, soda. Be alert to foods with hidden sugar, such as salad dressings or ketchup. Avoid alcohol, chocolate, cakes and carbonated beverages.

56. Eat plain yogurt.

57. Consider taking probiotics in a supplement form.

58. Enzyme supplements are available that are made specifically to fight yeast.

59. Replace your regular salt with Celtic salt or kosher salt.

60. **Adrenal Cleanse:** Adrenal fatigue, also known as adrenal burn-out, impacts many women suffering with infertility. If you are having trouble getting pregnant, this could be one of the not-so-obvious and sometimes difficult to diagnose reasons behind your infertility. The adrenals are a very important to your fertility because they are part of the endocrine system, which is responsible for producing and balancing more than 50 hormones in your body.

When the adrenals are weak or not working at full capacity, the body's entire endocrine system and hormones can become imbalanced.

Adrenal burn-out occurs when the adrenals are stressed and pushed to the point where they begin producing excessive amounts of cortisol and adrenaline, which results in progesterone in the body producing too many stress hormones.

The adrenals become too sluggish, and then the other endocrine glands are not signaled to release their hormones, which results in the entire communication system in the endocrine glands breaking down.

Emotional trauma, living in a constant state of fight or flight, chemical toxins, lack of sleep, anxiety, stress, depression, poor diet, infections, and some prescription drugs, can all cause adrenal burn-out.

If the adrenals are exhausted, you may not produce enough progesterone, which is the pro-gestational hormone needed to get pregnant and carry a pregnancy to term.

Here are some ways to help strengthen your adrenals:

61. Take a Vitamin C supplement. The adrenal gland uses vitamin C at a higher rate than other cells in the body.

62. Don't let your blood sugar levels get too low. Eat regular meals and never skip breakfast. Keep your blood sugar levels normal by eating healthy foods throughout the day.

63. Stop drinking coffee or drink no more than one cup of coffee a day. Caffeine depletes the body of B vitamins, which the adrenals need. Stop trying to energize and push your body by drinking another cup of coffee. Instead, eat fruits and vegetables that will provide your body with healthy forms of energy.

64. Drink lots of high-quality water.

65. Consider taking a Vitamin B complex, Vitamin E and an adrenal gland supplement.

66. A high-quality liquid trace mineral supplement can help support the adrenal glands. Note: Although you may want to drastically reduce your intake of this supplement once you are pregnant, or consult with a doctor on the levels of minerals that are safe and healthy to take during pregnancy.

67. Make lifestyle changes that reduce stress in your life. Do you need to change jobs? Relocate? Take a hard and honest look at the way you live your daily life. Start including more activities in your life that eliminate stress and reduce a fight-or-flight way of living. These include: deep breathing, massage, daily walks by a lake, ocean or in a beautiful park.

Consider more time for prayer, journal writing, and positive visualization.

68. Foods that help adrenals include spinach, garlic, onions, green leafy vegetables and brown rice.

69. Almonds and cashews, which are high in magnesium, are very healthy for the adrenal system.

70. Eat more seeds, such as sunflower and pumpkin seeds.

71. Avoid white flour products, soda, sugary fruit juices or anything that makes blood sugar levels rise rapidly.

72. Alternative health therapies, such as applied kinesiology, myofascial release, and craniosacral therapy can restore a weakened adrenal system.

73. Getting more sleep and better sleep can help restore the adrenal glands. So, go to bed earlier, preferably aim for a 9 to 10 o'clock bedtime, and try to stop all technology and electronic stimulation about an hour before bed for a better quality sleep.

74. Sea salt, celtic salt or regular salt in moderate amounts can help the adrenal system provided that you don't suffer from high-blood pressure.

75. Healthy fats like olive oil, coconut oil, ground flax seed or flax seed oil are excellent for burnt-out and exhausted adrenals.

76. Adrenal exhaustion can sometimes be caused by hidden food allergies. Find out if you are allergic to wheat, corn or dairy products.

77. A Colon Cleanse: Cleansing your colon can significantly improve your overall health and fertility. A colon that is diseased, inflamed or full of yeast, mold, fungus or parasites can cause a general malaise in the body and lower the body's pH balance, making it more acidic – and acid creates a hostile environment for reproductive health.

A colon that is weighed down by years of buildup can also press on the uterus and surrounding reproductive organs. Those who have undergone colon cleanses will attest to the dramatic improvements in how they feel afterwards.

By ridding your body of decaying matter, you could very well be turning back the hands of time. Colon cleansing, sometimes called colon hydrotherapy, can rid the body of chemicals and toxins that affect the egg and sperm.

Colonic irrigation and herbal cleansings help remove toxins, parasites and mucus that have built up in the colon. By flushing out impacted waste, passing stool is easier and transit times are improved. Removing impurities goes a long way in helping the body absorb nutrients, and enhancing energy levels.

Some doctors believe that poor bowel management is at the root of many health problems, and many diseases are a result of toxins built-up in the intestinal tract that are not eliminated. A digestive tract that has a build-up of unhealthy, slow moving foods that stick to the intestinal walls result in an overburdened colon full of decaying fecal matter and foods are acid-forming.

Yeasts, molds, fungus, bacteria, parasites and fecal materal can then enter the blood stream, causing what is known as leaky bowel syndrome. This results in a reduction of nutrients the body is able to absorb, and in turn impacts fertility.

Have your colon cleansed, at a licensed, reputable establishment with a long-time track record.

This can be an uncomfortable process, but in cleaning out your colon, you will be bringing new youth to your body.

You can also clean your colon with colon cleansing products available online, or at a natural foods store or supermarket.

Note: once there is even a chance that you are pregnant, stop all colon cleanses. This is something to be done only BEFORE there is any chance you are pregnant. If there is any possibility that you are pregnant, do not continue with any type of colon cleanse.

Here are some other ways to cleanse and detoxify your colon:

78. Foods that help keep the colon clean include apples, blackberries, blueberries, raspberries, figs, dates, avocados, spinach, Swiss chard, oatmeal, flax, and chickpeas.

79. Foods to avoid include sugar, white flour, and hormone/antibiotic-filled meats that assault the body.

80. Fennel and garlic are known to kill bacteria and parasites in the colon, thus improving colon function.

81. Cayenne pepper and garlic are also known colon cleansers.

82. Flaxseeds and psyllium husk seeds help clean the colon.

83. Herbs like Slippery Elm and Cascara Sagrada also are used in many colon detoxification cleanses.

84. Eat large amounts of fiber.

85. Ginger and garlic can help with healthy bowel movements, along with some olive oil in the morning. Leafy greens and healthy fibers can also aid in elimination.

86. Apples and carrots, which contain a large amount of water, go far in cleansing the colon.

87. Consider juicing apples, carrots, spinach, and other green vegetables as a way to help cleanse the colon.

88. Be aware of your bowel movements. Make sure you are having at least one healthy bowel movement a day. Don't hold in a bowel movement if you feel it coming.

89. Drink lemon, honey or maple syrup and cayenne pepper several times a day. Drink with or without food for several days as a way to cleanse the colon.

90. Reduce the amount of processed foods, fast foods, pizza and foods with additives that you eat.

91. While detoxifying your colon, start taking probiotics as a way to replenish your intestinal flora.

92. Eat a diet with a lot of high fiber vegetables, such as dark leafy greens,

93. Drink a lot of high-quality water each day. Inadequate hydration can lead to a build-up of toxins in the colon.

94. Juice or make a drink with vegetables daily.

95. Include essential fatty acids in your diet, such as ground flax seed, evening primrose oil, cod liver oil and coconut oil.

96. Eat foods rich in healthy fats, such as avocados, olive oil and nuts.

97. Include more olive oil in your diet, because it reduces bile acid and increase enzymes that regulate cell turn over in the lining of the intestines.

98. In Chinese medicine, the colon is one of the two organs in the metal element, and has the function of eliminating what is unnecessary or toxic in our bodies. On the emotional level, the colon enables us to let go of the garbage directed at our bodies and spirit. To heal the colon, it is important to 'let go' of negative experiences that may have tainted our self-worth.

For issues that are unresolved, write them on paper and burn them, thus releasing their content. Breath slowly and deeply each day. As you breath, feel the negativity, impurity and pain leave your body, and breath in energized, purified air. If you are chronically constipated, it may be that you are having a hard time letting go of something in your life, such as a past hurt, rejection or trauma. Allow yourself to accept and be open to new experiences in your life. As much as you can, make room for new, transforming experiences in your life.

99. **Kidney Cleanse:** According to Chinese herbal medicine, one of the most common causes of infertility is a problem with or a deficiency in the kidney. In fact, in Chinese medicine, a kidney deficiency is the most common diagnosis in infertility.

In Chinese medicine, the kidney is considered the main root of our Qi (chi) which regulates reproduction and is considered the seat of procreation, the vitality center of the body. A weak Qi, or kidney function, affects the quality and development of eggs, and impacts the ovaries and uterus.

A kidney deficiency is often a result of poor diet and stress.

Here are various ways to cleanse and strengthen the kidney:

100. Make sure you are working on cleansing and detoxifying the liver, because a healthy, clean liver results in a healthy, strong kidney.

101. Find an acupuncturist who is experienced in working with kidney deficiency and its impact on fertility.

102. Stop all coffee or limit coffee intake to no more than a cup a day.

103. Avoid carbonated beverages, artificial sweeteners and excessive amounts of dairy products.

104. Limit red meat.

105. Reduce sugar and sodium in your diet. Stop potato chips, crackers, cheese spreads, deli meats and instant potato mixes.

106. Kidney problems are often the result of stress, chronic anger and shame, so it is important to release and free yourself from these feelings. Journal writing, prayer, forgiveness of yourself and others, are all steps that can begin the healing process.

107. Dandelion tea is known to help flush toxins from the kidney.

108. Cod liver oil contains high levels of Vitamin D that strengthen the kidneys.

109. Foods that regenerate the kidney include chestnuts, strawberries, walnuts, raspberries; black, kidney and mung beans, fennel, onions, beetroot, garlic, ginger, cloves, red bell peppers, cabbage, cauliflower, dandelion, blueberries, red grapes, and wild salmon.

110. Add lots of flaxseed, pumpkin, and sunflower seeds to your diet.

111. Walnuts and chestnuts enhance the kidney's function.

112. Spirulina, kelp, chlorella, and wheatgrass are good for the kidney.

113. Eat lots of asparagus and other deep green leafy vegetables.

114. The herb Nettle is known to strengthen the kidney.

115. Drink lots of water.

116. Limit alcohol intake. Do not overtax your kidney with too much alcohol.

117. Juice cabbage, parsley, cucumbers and ginger.

118. Eat more apples, cranberries, olive oil, and onions.

119. Stay away from high-sodium foods.

120. Milk thistle is a great nutrient for the kidney.

121. Staying hydrated is very important to flushing out toxins in the kidney.

122. Eat large amounts of watermelon for a few days.

123. A Chinese herbalist can provide herbal formulas to clean the kidney.

124. Burdock tea helps removes waste from the kidneys.

125. Dandelion tea is known to help cleanse the kidneys.

126. Ginger root and turmeric tea is good for the kidneys and can be made by boiling some turmeric powder with peeled ginger root.

127. Grapes and cranberries. Grapes help flush uric acid and other waste products from the kidney. Cranberries contain quinine, which the liver converts to hippuric acid, which in turns helps remove urea and uric acid from the kidneys.

128. Apples are often used as a home remedy for kidney stones.

129. Garlic is a natural diuretic that helps flush out kidneys.

130. Cucumbers are a natural diuretic that can dissolve kidney and bladder stones.

131. Onions can help pass kidney stones.

132. Kidney beans and peas contain arginine, an amino acid that helps cleanse the kidney of ammonia.

133. Make sure you are getting enough Vitamin C, Vitamin E, calcium and B-6.

134. Keep your blood pressure, blood glucose level, and cholesterol levels in healthy ranges, so your kidneys are not overtaxed.

135. According to natural healers, the emotion that seems to impact the kidney the most is fear. Some believe that chronic fear and anxiety in childhood impacts the health of the kidneys later in life. To release fear, begin to embrace your life with courage. Welcome life! Do not push it away or hid from it. In Chinese medicine, the ability to use our will power to express our unique creativity is also dependent on good kidney energy. With a strong kidney qi, we will have the resolve to overcome fear and pursue goals. A weak kidney results in a shaky sense of purpose and one who is easily distracted.

Feeling stuck and not letting go is also sometimes the emotional root of kidney disease. The kidneys can store deep sadness, which can in turn result in illness. It is important to work on letting go of anger, fear, and traumatic, painful memories. Bring balance into your life in whenever way you can. Enjoy natural beauty and lots of rest. Spend more time enjoying natural bodies of water, such as lakes, oceans, and rivers. Keep a bowl of water with flowers nearby.

136. Get a foot massage. Ask the massage therapist to stimulate and massage the kidney point on the foot that will revitalize the kidney qi.

137. **Parasite Cleanse:** Another facet of cleansing is eliminating parasites in your body. Parasites can impact hormone levels and some nutritionists feel that parasites can also weaken a man's sperm quality.

Symptoms of parasites include brain fog or mental fuzziness, toe fungus or athletes foot, constant illness, rectal itching, especially at night, endometriosis, anxiety and depression.

Sleep problems, immune disorders, teeth grinding, eczema, hives, and chronic fatigue can also be the result of parasites.

Common tests that can discover whether or not you have parasites include a comprehensive digestive stool analysis, candida testing and a gastric acid self-test. Doctors can also test for parasites through x-rays.

To avoid getting parasites, do not eat raw fish or sushi and be sure to cook all fish very well. Avoid undercooked meat. Wash all fruits and vegetables thoroughly. Be very careful when eating at salad bars.

Do not let animals lick you in the face or mouth. Be aware of foods you eat when you visit other countries.

Health food stores and various health-related web sites have various parasite cleanses to choose from, and this is often a first and best step to rid the body of parasites. Make sure to drink lots of water while cleansing.

Along with doing a parasite cleanse, here are some tips on ridding your body of parasites:

138. Pineapple is an effective agent in ridding the body of parasites. Pineapple contains the digestive enzyme bromelain that can help clear tapeworms.

139. The probiotics in yogurt are also known to kill parasites.

140. Avoid sugar. Parasites are known to feed off sugar—so the less that is in your system, the less they are able to flourish within your body.

141. Avoid or reduce white flour products.

142. Apple cider vinegar, which is high in B-vitamins, can help neutralize the body's pH balance and improve digestion.

143. Probiotics can help restore gut bacteria wiped out by parasites. Do not take a probiotic, however, within an hour of taking apple cider vinegar.

144. Cinnamon is a natural remedy for parasites.

145. Include more garlic in your diet. Juice it, eat it, include it in your meals, whenever you can.

146. Olive oil can help remove parasite waste.

147. Trichomoniasis is a vaginal infection that is seen to play a role in infertility. Ask to be tested for this.

148. Chlorphyl can help eliminate parasites.

149. Papaya seeds are a natural method for removing parasites. Blend them with honey or coconut oil, as a parasite cleanse. Make sure to drink lots of water while cleansing.

150. Pumpkin seeds are effective in killing roundworms or tapeworms. Oven roast lightly. Try to eat on an empty stomach.

151. Eat pomegranates alone as they are known for destroying worms in the intestinal tract.

152. Cloves and turmeric can help fight parasites.

153. Sweet potatoes and squash can increase resistance to parasites because of their high Vitamin A content.

154. Raw onions and garlic provide sulfur containing amino acids that are anti-parasitic.

155. Thyme and thyme tea can help clear the body of parasites.

156. Cayenne pepper helps repel parasites.

157. A colonic irrigation, also known as a colon cleaning, can also help kill parasites.

158. **Uterine Cleanse:** You want to do everything possible to create the best and healthiest environment for your growing baby, and that means doing what is needed to create a healthy uterine lining for implantation of your embryos.

Conditions like hormonal imbalance, low circulation, or an unhealthy diet can impact the uterus. Other factors that impact the condition of the uterus include: stagnation of blood flow to the uterus, uterine fibroids, scar tissue from a cesarean, abdominal surgery, a D&C after a miscarriage, endometriosis, or a pelvic inflammatory disease caused by a sexually transmitted disease.

Here are some ways to cleanse and strengthen your uterus:

159. Goldenseal root cleanses the uterus.

160. Dong Quai, an herb, increases blood flow to the uterus and builds the uterine lining. It also tones and strengthens the uterus by regulating hormonal balance, improving uterine tone and is a blood tonic that helps circulation. It also relieves congestion and pain in the reproductive system.

161. Damiana, an herb, encourages circulation and blood supply to the uterus.

162. Red Raspberry Leaf or Red Raspberry Root has long been used as a uterine tonic to regulate and tone uterine muscles. It can be taken as a supplement or a tea.

163. Eat or juice dandelion leaves, spinach, beets, garlic and lemon.

164. Nettle Leaves is a uterine cleanser.

165. L-Arginine promotes synthesis of nitric oxide, which increases blood flow to the uterus and ovaries.

166. Eating foods rich in zinc can help strengthen the uterus. These include pumpkin seeds, sesame seeds and spinach.

167. Some health practitioners recommend propping one's legs up against a wall 15 minutes a day to encourage increased blood flow to the uterus.

168. Avoid soy and peas.

169. Acupuncture can help bring more blood to your uterus. Let your acupuncturist know you are working on fertility and would like to improve your circulation to your uterus.

170. Eat blood nourishing foods, such as spinach and dates.

171. Pomegranates and pomegranate juice can help build uterine lining.

172. Chinese medicine adheres to the belief that it is important to keep the uterus and belly warm while trying to get pregnant. They suggest not drinking or eating anything too cold, wearing socks and keeping one's feet warm at night. Do not go barefoot or wear flip-flops. However, this does not mean overheating your body with a water bottle or doing anything that could overheat a growing fetus.

173. Write a letter to your womb. Let whatever wants to be said come up and be said. Express whatever you are feeling, whether it is anger, fear or lack of self-love. Do not repress any of your feelings. Allow yourself the freedom to speak your truth, whatever it is.

174. Practice deep breathing into your uterus and repeat the affirmation: I receive, I receive, I receive. I receive my baby, I receive my baby, I receive my baby.

175. Your uterus deserves acknowledgement, respect and unconditional love. It needs to be told it is strong enough, good enough and worthy enough to receive a baby.

176. A Native American fertility tradition is to wear a long skirt with no underwear, and sit on the ground to release whatever wounds are within you into the earth. As you do this, imagine your womb is a beautiful flowering place full of energy and light. Let the earth's energy flow up to your uterus, so it can draw from the healing energy of the earth.

177. Pineapple contains a proteolytic enzyme called bromelain which reduces inflammation and breaks up proteins that prevent embryo implantation. Eating pineapple core a few days before and after an IVF cycle can help implantation. But stop eating pineapple immediately after any IVF or IUI or if you think if there is any chance you might be pregnant. While pineapple helps implantation, it is definitely not recommended for pregnancy.

178. Eat lots of blueberries. Research shows they contain anthocyanins that help maintain the lining of the uterus.

179. Brazil nuts contain selenium, that can thicken the uterine lining and help with implantation.

180. Foods with omega-3 fatty acids can improve blood flow to the uterus, such as salmon, flaxseed oil, pumpkin seeds, walnuts, and olive oil.

181. See a massage therapist who is familiar with massage to help increase circulation to the uterus and unblock the reproductive system. Look for a massage therapist experienced in deep tissue massage or massage that is used to clear blocked energy in the organs.

182. Acupressure, myofacial release and reflexology can also offer massage that brings blood and oxygen to the reproductive organs.

183. Ask your uterus these questions: have you ever felt judged? Blamed? Abused? What do you need to heal? What can I do to help you feel loved and nurtured? Write the answers that come up from within you.

184. Visualize your uterus as a cozy, warm, loving and safe place for your baby. Repeat, write and sing these affirmations:
-my uterus is healthy and just right for my baby
-my uterus welcomes my baby
-my uterus is a safe and welcoming place for my baby
-my uterus is a healing, balanced, and loving home for my baby
-I love you uterus. Thank you for taking good care of my baby.
-Uterus, you are enough. You are enough to hold my baby.
-Dear uterus, I honor and respect you.

185. Supplements recommended to help implantation include zinc, Vitamin C, selenium and iron.

186. Important To Note: herbs used to strengthen and cleanse your uterus must be stopped once there is any chance you are pregnant or while taking infertility medications.

187. **Blood Cleanse:** You want to cleanse your blood of toxins and chemicals as much as possible, because chemicals and toxins in your bloodstream can impact the health of your eggs and various organs that impact fertility.

Here are some ways to cleanse and detoxify your blood:

188. Chlorophyll is known to cleanse the blood of impurities.

189. Juice or eat cilantro, parsley and beets. Beet juice is a strong blood purifier.

190. Drink lemon and water

191. Burdock Root is revered by natural practitioners as one of the most effective blood cleansers and purifiers.It strengthens the liver and increases urination to help the kidneys remove toxins from the blood.

192. Yellow Dock Root enriches and purifies the blood

193. Dandelion promotes bile production that breaks down fats in the body, and destroys harmful microbes found in digested food that can enter the bloodstream.

194. Goji berries are a powerful antioxidant that alkalize the blood.

195. Consider digestive enzymes between meals or before bed

196. Red clover is a blood purifier.

197. Apple cider vinegar helps cleanse the blood.

198. Echinacea is known for enhancing the immune system and cleaning the blood of pathogens.

199. Drink lots of pure water

200. Garlic is a strong blood purifier. Juice it, eat it, crush cloves of garlic in water and drink it, or chew on raw garlic each day.

201. Turmeric purifies the blood

202. Teas made from Oregon Grape Root and Sarsaparilla Root rid the blood of waste products.

203. Broccoli, cabbage, cauliflower and watercress are all blood purifiers. Some recommend juicing cauliflower as a great way to clean your blood.

204. Parsley is a natural blood cleanser.

205. Cayenne pepper improves the circulatory system by cleaning out the channels that the blood flows through.

206. **A Lymph System Cleanse:** The lymph is a very important, but often overlooked, system in the body that impacts fertility. It is so important that some health practitioners believe that a clogged, sluggish, toxic lymph system accounts for many illnesses in the body.

The lymph system is a complex system of vessels and ducts that move fluid and toxins out of the body. A sluggish lymph system means the body is not disposing of waste properly. This affects fertility because the lymphatic system plays a key role in the circulation of hormones, and a stagnant lymphatic system can impact the feedback system of these hormones.

A cleansed lymph system can help revive sluggish, congested ovaries and reduce acid levels in the vagina.

Lack of exercise, a sedentary lifestyle, stress, chronic digestive imbalances, and a high-sodium diet, can make the lymphatic system sluggish and ineffective.

Symptoms of a sluggish lymph system include feeling tired and fatigued, getting sick a lot, being overweight, having fatty deposits of cellulite, acne, rashes, as well as having lots of food sensitivities and allergies. Some believe that fibromyalgia and chronic fatigue syndrome are a result of a clogged lymph system.

Here are some ways to cleanse the lymph system:

207. To help the flow of your lymph system, drink plenty of high-quality water each day. Staying well hydrated is key to a healthy lymph system.

208. Eliminate, as much as you can, sugar, soda and fruit juices from your diet.

209. Always remember that the lymph system has no pump, so it is up to you to help keep your lymph flowing by drinking lots of water and moving your body. Exercises such as jumping on a mini-trampoline, dancing, walking or swimming are helpful. Jumping helps the lymphatic circulation by stimulating the millions of one-way valves in the system. If you are laid up due to a surgery or illness, it is important to find ways to move the lymph system, such as a lymph massage of a self-massage.

210. Do deep breathing exercises.

211. Eat lots of green vegetables to purify the blood and lymph.

212. Essential fatty acids are important to the lymph. Walnuts and flaxseeds give the lymph system the fatty acids it needs. Almonds, sunflower seeds, pumpkin seeds, Brazil nuts, coconut oil and flaxseed oil also provide essential fatty acid.

213. Use a natural bristle brush to brush your skin in circular motions, upward from the feet to the torso, before showering.

214. Avoid processed foods that have artificial preservatives, flavors, colors, stabilizers, which includes many packaged and fast foods. These can also include hot dogs, canned foods, cereals, packaged dinners and luncheon meats.

215. Avoid fatty foods and white breads.

216. Raw fruit is a powerful lymph cleanser.

217. Cranberries and cranberry juice can also help emulsify fat in the lymph system.

218. Foods that help the lymph system include beets, onions, garlic, avocados, seaweed, kelp, kombu, kale, radish and mustard greens.

219. Juice one green drink a day.

220. Eat lots of citrus fruits, like lemons and limes.

221. Take chlorophyll to help purify your lymph system.

222. Consider an apple cider vinegar cleanse that combines honey, garlic and apple cider in a blender.

223. Herbs such as Echinacea, Goldenseal and Astragalus can lessen congestion and swelling in the lymphatic system.

224. One of the ways to cleanse your lymph system is a lymphatic massage, sometimes called manual lymphatic drainage.

Lymph massage is a very gentle form of deep tissue massage that moves the lymph under your skin, freeing trapped toxins and improves lymph flow in the body. It combines a gentle pressure with soft pumping movements in the direction of the lymph nodes in the body. You can find this type of practitioner by searching 'lymphatic drainage massage with your city/town/' or by searching holistic practitioners in your area, who might be able to direct you to someone who does this type of massage.

Here are more ways to cleanse your lymph system:

225. Massaging under your arms can be helpful in relieving congestion. Place your fingertips under your armpit. Then gently push inward, towards the center of your body. Repeat this circular motion.

226. Acupuncture is very helpful to the lymph system.

227. Drink a cup of red clover tea each day.

228. Laugh from your belly, which helps pump your lymphatic system.

229. Avoid white flour products, white rice, bread and pasta, as much as possible.

230. Include bananas, raisins, dates, spinach and orange juice.

231. Sip hot water throughout the day.

232. Beets are healthy for the lymph system.

233. Cayenne pepper can boost a sluggish lymph system and reduce mucous congestion.

234. Stop using underarm deodorants that contain aluminium and clog the natural excretion of toxins from the lymph system.

235. Stop wearing tight bras.

236. Letting yourself feel your congested emotions encourages natural detoxification of the lymph system. Allow yourself to feel. Let yourself express your grief through crying, moving anger out of your body, talking, writing or whatever way your body chooses. Honor and express your emotions.

237. **Thyroid Cleanse:** Your thyroid is a key organ that impacts your fertility.

To keep your thyroid healthy:

238. As much as possible, eliminate gluten from your diet.

239. Alkalize your body as much as possible, through green vegetables, green drinks and green smoothies.

240. Drink warm lemon water throughout the day to loosen toxins in the digestive system.

241. Foods that can help the thyroid include: Spirulina, Brazil nuts, sunflower seeds, black walnuts.

242. Iodized table salt

243. Chlorophyl and coconut oil are known to strengthen the thyroid.

244. Avoid all soy products

245. Herbs to consider include Irish moss and Kelp.

246. **Balancing Your Hormones and Improving the Quality of Your Eggs:** If our hormones are not balanced, our fertility is compromised on every level. Our hormones, produced by our glands and tissues, are chemical communicators that deliver messages to our body. These messages are then released into our blood, where they travel to other tissues and send signals initiating various activities within our body and brain.

247. Our hormones are impacted by stress, fluid changes in the body, vitamin and mineral levels, infections, exposure to environmental toxins and body fat. Blood sugar imbalances, a toxic liver, folic acid deficiency, inflammation in the ovaries, breast and joints, and unhealthy gut flora can all be a result of unbalanced hormones.

248. Be alert to Other symptoms of a hormonal imbalance can include insomnia, headaches, migraines, anxiety, foggy thinking, hot flashes, mood swings, thinning hair, bloating, rapid heartbeat, and allergies. Our hormones are impacted by stress, fluid changes in the body, vitamin and mineral levels, infection and exposure to environmental toxins and body fat.

It is important to support and strengthen the entire endocrine system. Hormones are coordinated by this system, which includes the hypothalamus, pituitary gland, adrenal gland, thyroid, parathyroid, pancreas, pineal gland, thymus and ovaries. The foods you eat, the stress levels you experience, the chemicals in your environment, all impact the endocrine system, and in turn, your hormones.

Progesterone is a key hormone in fertility and you want to do whatever you can to make sure you have adequate progesterone levels in your body.

Progesterone plays an important role in conception and maintaining a healthy pregnancy. It works to balance the effects of estrogen.
It helps maintain the lining of the uterus, which makes it possible for a fertilized egg to attach and survive.

It also makes cervical mucous accessible to the sperm, preventing immune rejection of the developing baby and normalizes blood clotting. Progesterone is produced by the corpus luteum in the ovaries and by the adrenal glands.

One of the main causes of a progesterone defiency is too much estrogen in the body. Estrogen dominance is extremely dangerous to one's fertility. It can result from eating a lot of commercially raised meat and dairy products that contain large amounts of estrogen. Chemicals called xenoestrogens are often in these food sources and they mimic the hormone estrogen and disrupt the delicate balance between estrogen and progesterone. Other excess hormones and hormone-like substances found in our environment, food and water also impact progesterone levels in the body. Pollution, stress, processed foods, soy products, and endometriosis, can cause an overload of estrogen. Allergies like asthma, hives, dry eyes, weight gain, irregular periods, and foggy thinking are symptoms of estrogen dominance.

A low thyroid, recurrent early miscarriages, sleep disturbances, and heart palpitations, can sometimes be symptoms of progesterone deficiency.

Other hormones important to fertility include estradiol, or estrogen, that are produced by the follicles and corpus luteum, also known as the remnant egg sac in the ovaries. The luteinizing hormone, known as the LH surge, produced in the anterior pituitary gland, triggers ovulation and the development of the corpus luteum.

It works in conjunction with the follicle stimulating hormone (FSH) that is also released and synthesized by the anterior pituitary gland. The FSH hormone regulates the reproductive process and signals the follicles in the ovary to begin maturing in preparation for ovulation.

Tests that can track your hormone levels include progesterone, estradiol, FSH, LH, prolactin, testosterone, sex hormone binding globulin, glucose tolerance test, thyroid panel and a blood lipid panel.

Here are some ways to balance and maintain healthy fertility hormone levels in your body:

249. Reduce your exposure to xenohormones, which can be found in car exhaust, plastics, solvents, adhesives, pesticides, and emulsifiers found in soap and cosmetics and PCD's from industrial waste.

250. Consider the herb Chaste Tree Berry, also known as Vitex Extract, that can balance hormones and strengthen the pituitary and ovary glands. This herb can correct hormonal communication in the body and hormonal problems at their source.

251. Progesterone shots. You may want to talk to your doctor about progesterone shots if you had recurrent miscarriages or just want help maintaining your pregnancy. This is something to consider requesting if your doctor has not initiated it and if you exhibit the symptoms of a progesterone deficiency.

252. Natural progesterone cream. Check with your doctor and discuss the amount to use.

253. Vitamin B6 is known to help maintain optimal levels of progesterone and is key in progesterone production. Vitamin B also helps the liver break down estrogen. Food sources of Vitamin B6 can be found in walnuts, lean red meat, poultry, bananas, spinach, and potatoes.

254. Turmeric, thyme and oregano are all considered helpful in raising progesterone levels.

255. Vitamin C is known to considerably increase progesterone production.

256. Zinc is key for producing adequate levels of progesterone in the body. That is because Zinc is a mineral that prompts the pituitary gland to release follicle stimulating hormones, which in turn promote ovulation and stimulate the ovaries to produce estrogen and progesterone.

Along with a zinc supplement, natural sources of zinc include lean red meats, wheat germ, chickpeas, pumpkin and squash seeds, watermelon and dark chocolate.

257. Practice stress-reduction techniques, as stress can considerably reduce progesterone levels in the body.

258. Do you have low cholesterol? This can mean you are not making enough pregnenolone, which is used to make progesterone.

259. Are your adrenals healthy? They house DHEA that is essential to the production of progesterone. One way to improve your adrenal health is to improve your natural circadian rhythm and get more sleep.

260. Maintain a healthy digestive tract. If you have a damaged digestive tract, you won't have the raw materials within your body to absorb the nutrients in your food that helps the body produce hormones.

261. You may want to consider testing for parasites, candida, or pathogens which can impact your hormonal balance.

262. Maca, a root vegetable in the radish family, can balance hormones and nourish and balance the endocrine system. It protects the body from stress damage. Maca is a nutritionally dense super food that contains high amounts of minerals, vitamins, enzymes and all of the essential amino acids. Maca also stimulates and nourishes the hypothalamus and pituitary glands, which are the "master glands" of the body. It is available in powder form or capsules,

263. Coconut oil stimulates the thyroid and provides omega-3's that help balance hormones. Other healthy fats essential to hormone health include flax oil, evening primrose oil and olive oil.

264. Magnesium is known to break down excessive estrogens in the system and assist in balancing hormones. Kelp and cashews are rich in magnesium. Other sources of magnesium include black beans, spinach, okra, watermelon seeds, sunflower, pumpkin seeds and squash seeds.

265. Garlic is an important nutrient for the endocrine system.

266. Ginkgo and ginseng help regulate hormones

267. Consider supplements such as Vitamin C and Vitamin B.

268. Getting more sleep helps balance hormones.

269. Flaxseed contains lignans and fiber, which help remove excess estrogen from the body.

270. If you think you are overweight, consider trying to lose some of the weight to help your hormonal system.

271. Red Clover, an herb, protects the body from xenohormones.

272. Black Cohosh, an herb, is well-known for its effect on hormone functioning.

273. Do a liver cleanse. The liver plays a key role in to hormonal balance. Milk thistle, dandelion leaf and burdock root are all potent liver cleansers.

274. Royal jelly is rich in amino acids and contains acetylcholine, which is needed to transmit nerve messages from cell to cell.

275. Ashwagandha root supports endocrine system function and helps to regulate hormones.

276. Be aware of chemicals in your diet, water, and environment that can throw your hormones out of balance.

277. Drink only filtered water. Avoid water with fluoride. Fluoride is known to weaken the thyroid, one of the key organs responsible for your hormones.

278. Be aware of products that may contain aluminium, including deodorants, anti-perspirants, and cosmetics.

279. Be careful of meats coated with nitrate salts.

280. Do not eat foods from plastic containers. Whenever possible, use glass and stainless steel.

281. Avoid vegetable oil, canola oil, soybean oil, margarine, shortening and other chemically altered fats.

282. Drink whole milk, not skim milk

283. Licorice is a hormone balancer.

284. Natural sources of iodine can help regulate hormones. These include kelp, cranberries and strawberries.

285. Improve indoor air-quality with plants.

286. Limit caffeine.

287. Other supplements to consider for hormonal balance include calcium, Vitamin E and grapeseed extract.

288. Address your hormonal imbalance on the emotional level. Are you feeling trapped? Unloved? Stuck? Angry? Are you living in a way that is true to who you are? Let your body tell you why your hormones are imbalanced.

Foods To Help Balance Hormones:

289. Pumpkin seeds and Brazil nuts.

290. Avocados and acai

291. Spinach, kale, parsley, broccoli, asparagus and other leafy greens.

292. Sweet peppers.

293. Pears and peaches are known to help regulate hormones. They are used often in traditional Chinese medicine.

294. Shiitake and reishi mushrooms, chia seeds, seaweed and spirulina.

295. Avocados block estrogen absorption and promote progesterone production.

296. **How to Improve Your Egg Quality:** Good news—you can improve the health and quality of your eggs.

In the past, we were told we were all born with a certain number of egg cells that run out as we age. We were led to believe that egg cells were the only cells in the body that did not regenerate, but instead were a finite number. We are finding out THIS IS JUST NOT TRUE. Recent research has shown that women can produce new eggs throughout their reproductive years.

You may have been told that your eggs are not healthy or that your eggs are too old.

Here's the great news: there is much you can do to enhance the health of your eggs. It was commonly believed that the only factor that determined egg health and quality was age. Several new studies have shown that stress, hormones and environmental toxins all impact our egg health. Your egg's health is a key cornerstone of a healthy fertility, because the health of your eggs can affect whether or not fertilization, implantation and ultimately a healthy pregnancy and birth will occur.

Here are some things you can do to improve your egg health:

296. Coenzyme Q10: Coenzyme Q10 is an excellent way to improve the quality and energy within your eggs. In several studies, the supplement Coenzyme Q10 has been shown to improve egg quality. It boosts energy production in the oocytes, which are cells in the ovary. Providing additional energy in the form of Coenzyme Q10 is needed when there is decreased energy production in the ovaries due to aging. It is also a source of fuel for the mitochondria, which produces energy within the cells and with age, can begin to weaken.
Along with taking a Coenzyme Q10 supplement, natural sources of CoQ10 include almonds, spinach, sardines, broccoli, strawberries, and walnuts.

297. Green Tea: Green Tea contains hypoxanthine which provides follicular fluid that helps eggs mature, along with polyphenols that are powerful antioxidants that prevent chromosomal abnormalities, and repair oxidative damage within the body. However, green tea can reduce the body's absorption of folic acid, so you may want to increase your dosage of folic acid at the same time.

298. Start eating foods high in antioxidants that will protect your eggs from free radical damage. Free radicals can damage both the egg cell health and the cell's DNA. Foods high in antioxidants that can combat free radicals include blueberries, cranberries, garlic, Granny apples, artichokes, spinach, kale, broccoli, plums, walnuts, and oregano.

299. Include Maca in your diet, which is a root-like cruciferous vegetable and the only plant known in the world that can grow and thrive at a high altitude in harsh weather. Maca contains 31 different minerals and 60 different phytonutrients. It nourishes the endocrine system, aids the pituitary, adrenal and thyroid glands, and helps balance hormones and increases energy and stamina in the body.

Maca controls estrogen levels in the body, which is very important because if estrogen levels are too high or low, it can prevent a woman from becoming pregnant or carrying full term. Excess estrogen levels can also cause progesterone levels to become low.

Make sure that when you purchase Maca, it contains the root, not just leaves and stem. Once, you are pregnant, you need to stop Maca immediately—it is to be taken only to prepare your body to become pregnant.

300. L-Arginine is an amino acid that has been shown to increase ovarian response, endometrial receptivity and pregnancy rates.

301. Royal Jelly

302. Omega-E fatty acid

303. New research has shown that melatonin can improve egg quality. Consider taking a melatonin supplement, because new research has shown that the hormone melatonin may help improve egg quality.

Supplements to Consider:

304. Vitamin B

305. DHEA

306. Spirulina

307. Red raspberry leaf

308. Flaxseed

309. Coconut oil

310. Olive oil

311. Grapeseed extract

312. Pomegranate

313. Kelp

314. Bee pollen

315. Improve the blood flow and oxygenation to your ovaries. Oxygen rich blood flow to the ovaries is essential for good egg health. A lack of good blood flow can be due to lack of exercise, dehydration and thick blood. To increase blood flow to the ovaries, drink at least 8 glasses of pure, high-quality water each day. Make sure the water is NOT bottled in plastic. Do light exercise, such as walking. Massage your uterus and ovaries. You might want to look for a massage therapist experienced in abdomen massage

316. Hormonal balance is key to proper egg health and cleansing your system of excess hormones can help. You can do this by doing a liver cleanse, especially if you suffer from an overabundance of estrogen.

317. Work on improving your uterine health. Some herbs that can help include Burdock Root, Milk Thistle Seed, Dandelion Root, Yellow Dock Root, Licorice Root and Goldenseal Root to cleanse the uterus.

318. If your FSH levels are high, consider Vitex, a shrub native to Greece and Italy whose berries have been used in herbal medicine for centuries. Vitex has an amazing ability to balance fertility hormones and is considered one of the most useful herbs in fertility. It helps support and regulate the pituitary gland, inhibits follicle-stimulating hormones, lengthens the luteal phase, and increases progesterone levels.

319. Reduce stress as much as you can in your life.

320. In Chinese medicine, ovarian health is linked to kidney health. Do a kidney cleanse and eat foods that support and strengthen your kidney.

321. Start acupuncture treatments once, twice or three times a week.

322. Be aware of the two most common allergens that can impact your body, gluten and dairy.

323. Avoid environmental contaminants.

324. Avoid dietary fats.

325. Be aware of insulin levels and eat in a way that reduces blood sugar level spikes.

326. Avoid white flour products

327. Repeat affirmations like "my eggs are healthy and can create a beautiful baby."

Foods and Substances To Avoid:

328. To maximize your egg health, you want to reduce your exposure to xenohormones, which are substances not found in nature that have hormonal effects on the body. These toxic substances can be absorbed through the skin and build up in the body over time.

329. Sources of xenohormones include solvents and adhesives, including paint, varnish, nail polish and in dry cleaning, car exhaust, all plastics, meat from non-organic livestock, pesticides, herbicides and fungicides, emulsifiers in soap and cosmetics, bug sprays, lawn sprays, and pesticides.

330. Avoid cosmetics and soaps made with petrochemical emulsifiers.

331. Do not use mineral oil on your body. Do not microwave your food in plastic. Stop wearing polyester clothing.

332. Do not use air fresheners, fabric softeners, spermicide, feminine care products.

333. Avoid cigarettes, coffee, alcohol, sugar, non-organic meats and dairy products

334. Avoid soda

335. Avoid diet foods, processed foods, trans fats and GMO foods.

336. Do not eat corn

337. Very little to no gluten if possible

338. No soy

339. Avoid all monounsaturated fats

Foods To Enhance Your Egg Health and Quality

340. Broccoli, berries, dark leafy vegetables, salmon, pumpkin seeds

341. Sesame seeds

342. Turmeric

343. Dark green leafy vegetables, such as kale, spinach or chard

344. Start making your own super fertility smoothie, with ingredients like spinach, strawberries, spirulina, Maca Root, bee pollen, royal jelly, and flax seed.

345. **Be Aware of Electromagnetic Energy:** There is research that suggests that electromagnetic fields can reduce fertility. Don't get panicked about this, but just be aware of how much electromagnetic energy you come in contact with daily.

Here are some steps you can take to reduce your exposure to electromagnetic energy:

346. Take all electrical devices out of your bedroom, or at least unplug them before you go to sleep at night. Remove or unplug radios, TVs, stereos, alarm clocks and computers in your bedroom.

347. If you can, reduce your time in front of a computer. Surf the Internet only when you need to. Unplug your computer when not in use.

348. Keep your microwave unplugged and stand faraway from it while using it.

349. Reduce the time spent on your cell phone. Use your cell phone only for emergencies, and do not keep it in your pocket.

350. If you are using a cordless phone, change back to a standard fixed line when you are at home if you can.

351. For now, put away electric blankets.

352. Keep laptops off your body.

353. Unplug electrical appliances while not in use.

354. Use manual toothbrushes, not electric. As much as possible, do things manually—also known as the old-fashioned way—at least for now. Whenever you can, reduce your time on devices that are wireless.

While we need these modern conveniences, reduce your time near them as much as possible. Instead, surround your body with as much natural forms of energy as possible, such sunlight.

355. **Get More Sleep:** Many studies are now suggesting that not getting enough sleep can impact a woman's fertility because sleep has a powerful influence on the body's hormonal system. Those who don't get enough sleep have higher levels of the stress hormone cortisol and adrenocorticotropic, which can suppress a healthy fertility cycle.

Here are some ways to enjoy better sleep:

356. Try to get on a regular sleep schedule. No more staying up until 11:30 watching TV or surfing the Internet. If possible, try for a 8, 9 or 10 o'clock bedtime, which gives your body plenty of pre-midnight sleep time.

357. Some believe that one hour of sleep before midnight is worth two hours after, meaning that the body benefits from pre-midnight sleep enormously Think of our ancestors, who went to bed soon after the sun set. Their body clocks aligned with the natural world, allowing them maximum rest and rejuvenation.

358. The body reportedly needs seven to nine hours of sleep a night. Chart your sleep schedule to see if you are within this range. The goal should be getting to bed earlier to ensure more pre-midnight sleep time, and a regular sleep schedule that eliminates any chance that your body might be suffering from sleep deprivation.

359. Exercising lightly and getting enough sunlight is reported to help encourage healthy sleep patterns. Do not drink anything caffeinated in the afternoon. Stay on a relatively predictable bedtime schedule.

360. Avoid watching TV late at night, or checking e-mail, which can be overstimulating. Some studies have shown that those who consume electronic media just before bedtime experience lower-quality sleep.

361. To experience higher quality and deeper sleep, consider relaxing activities before bed such as reading, taking a bath, knitting, listening to soothing music, doing a jigsaw puzzle, or drawing or sketching in bed. For me, prayer is my most relaxing bedtime routine.

362. Keep your bedroom as dark as possible. A better night's sleep is achieved in total darkness. Block your windows or get room darkening shades. Light at night can impact your pineal gland. Remove or unplug anything in your room that emits light, such as night lights, clock radios or computers. Do not keep chargers in your bedroom.

363. **Be Aware Of The Chemicals In Your Environment:** We all know that toxins and chemicals in our environment are not good for us, and while it is useless to obsess about this or try to control every element of this, there are some things that you can do to reduce the amount of chemical toxins that enter your system while you are trying to conceive. A note of caution here: don't get too paranoid. Despite the pollution in our environment, millions of babies are born every day in all parts of the world, smog filled or not. The human body is strong and can handle a lot—worrying about what is out of your control won't do you any good right now. Your body can handle more than you probably can imagine, and you are not a victim of even the most polluted environment. But when it is in your realm of control, do what you can do to keep your body chemical-free. Think about what you touch and take into your body that is within your realm of control.

Here are some ways to reduce the toxins that enter your system:

364. Try not to purchase soaps and cleaning products with the chemical triclocarban, or TCC in it.

365. Try to avoid using deodorant when you can, and if you feel it necessary, stick to a natural, aluminium-free deodorant.

366. Use regular soap, not anti-bacterial.

367. Buy natural cleaning products and laundry detergent.

368. Just for now, stop dyeing your hair or using nail polish.

369. Avoid products with perfluorooctanoate (PFOA) and perfluorooctane sulfonate (PFOS) that are used to manufacture Teflon non-stick coatings and is in some personal care products. Products known to contain these chemicals include carpet and fabric protectors, microwave popcorn bags and stain-proof clothing.

370. Avoid Bisphenol or (BPA) when possible. It is used in plastic water bottles, plastic microwavable plates and utensils, tooth sealants, and soda cans.

371. Phthalate is a compound used in perfumes, cosmetics and hairsprays. For now, stop using these products.

372. Buy bottled water or put a filter on your tap water at home. You may even want to consider a filter for the water you shower and cook with.

373. Avoid painting or being around paint while pregnant.

374. Avoid lawn, plant, gardening or insect pesticides.

375. Be aware of dry cleaning chemicals and do not have clothes dry-cleaned at this time.

376. Be weary of super strength cleaners. When possible, use homemade or natural cleaners. If you do use strong cleaners, wear gloves whenever possible to avoid the chemical seeping into your skin.

377. Avoid carpet cleaners and air fresheners if you can.

378. Avoid smelling fumes from household cleaners.

379. Beware of plastics. Don't microwave and eat from anything plastic while trying to conceive. If you purchase water in plastic jugs, try whenever possible to transfer the water to a glass jug. Plastics can seep into your system and impact your immune system. Do not purchase foods that have to be microwaved in plastic.

380. Buy an air purifier for your home.

381. Stop using cleaning products with ingredients you cannot identify. Buy only natural cleaning products, with ingredients you can pronounce and understand.

382. Just for now, stop using all chemical products on your hair and nails.

383. To remove environmental toxins from your body, consider one or more of the following: a liver cleanse, colon cleanse, kidney cleanse, heavy metal cleanse, parasite and/or yeast.

384. Find a professional in your area that offers a bio cleanse ionic foot bath, which is an effective way to remove toxins from the body. Some companies sell foot pads that can be used to detox and remove toxins.

385. Put more household plants in your house to help filter toxins from the air, or consider a HEPA filter for your home.

386. Stay aware of chemicals that you ingest, smell, or put on your skin and can enter your body.

387. Get More Sunlight: Both you and your husband/male partner should spend 15 to 30 minutes each day outside in sunlight, as some studies have shown that lack of sunlight can cause a deficiency in Vitamin D, which impacts infertility.

Take walks, or just put some chairs outside and sit for 20 minutes. Many studies have revealed that lack of sunlight can cause male infertility. Exposure to sunlight also stimulates the pineal gland, which increases serotonin, a chemical that produces good feelings in the brain.

388. Drink Lots of Good-Quality Water: When trying to conceive, drink lots of high-quality, filtered water. Some recommend 8-10 glasses of water a day or more. Water is critical because 75 percent of our body is made up of water. A water deficiency can impact the liver and kidney.

389. Deep Breath: Deep breathing helps your body release toxins, reduce anxiety levels, reduce inflammation, improve digestion and help you feel more relaxed. At least once or twice a day, spend some time consciously deep breathing. Breath through your nose down into your belly, and then exhale through your mouth.

Deep breathing also helps release endorphins and bring fresh oxygen to your cells. Schedule a specific time for deep breathing. You want to get into the habit of doing some deep breathing at the same time everyday, so it becomes part of your routine.

390. Enhance Your Cervical Mucous: Low cervical mucous can result from not enough water intake each day, poor circulation to the reproductive organs, hormonal imbalance and low progesterone levels.

Conditions That Might Be Threatening Your Fertility: Some of these conditions could be among the causes of your infertility.

391. Do You Have An Iron Deficiency?: Some studies have found a link between low iron intake and infertility. Low iron, or anemia, can increase the body's risk for being unable to produce healthy eggs. This is because a lack of iron can cause anovulation, or lack of ovulation and in turn, poor egg health. Being low in iron can cause eggs stored in the ovaries to be weak and unviable.

A lack of iron in the body also results in an insufficient number of red blood cells, which are responsible for delivering oxygen to the ovaries and uterus. Ask your physician for a test to see if you are anemic or low in iron. You may want to consider taking a high-quality iron supplement, either in capsule or liquid form, or a multivitamin that has iron in it.

Some studies have shown that it is best to take a vegetable based iron, rather than animal based. Eat more foods high in iron. These include spinach, beets, molasses, pumpkin seeds, asparagus.

Other iron rich foods include:

• Kale, broccoli, lean red meat, asparagus, parsley, kidney beans, lentils, apricots, and chicken.

• When you get pregnant, make sure your iron levels are sufficient throughout your pregnancy.

• Select an iron supplement that includes nutrients that help iron absorption, which are B12 (folic acid) and Vitamin C.

392. Consider Your Weight: Being overweight can cause your body to produce excess insulin, which stimulates the ovaries to produce testosterone male-like hormones. Being overweight can also cause hormonal irregularities and increase one's risk of miscarriage. So if you are overweight, do what you can do lose weight.

When I was trying to get pregnant for a second time, I was told that if I lost weight, my chances for conception would improve significantly. So I went to Friendly's, enjoyed a big five-scoop sundae with lots of hot fudge, and then I joined Weight Watchers. Over the course of seven months, I lost almost 50 pounds. I do believe this helped in my ultimately getting pregnant.

My diet consisted of a lean turkey meat sandwich with healthy bread and mustard, instead of mayonnaise. I also ate a lot of bowls of romaine lettuce and parsley as snacks at work.

I was sometimes called a 'rabbit' by my co-workers, and my nightly treat was sugar free, fat free pudding, although I stopped eating this the closer I got to the IVF procedure. I also ate a lot of Weight Watcher's garden vegetable soup. Cut down on white flour products, sugary juices, sodas and sugar. Write down everything you eat each day. Prepare snacks of cut and washed fruits and vegetables ahead of time each night, so you don't slip during the day.Find a support group or therapist to help if you relied on food to cope with emotional needs, such as loneliness or frustration.

393. Is Your Body's Energy Off Track?: Keeping the energy flow in your body on track is important to good health. In Chinese medicine, infertility is seen as an imbalance of the body's energy levels and that to heal one's infertility it is important to find the imbalances in the body, and then balance the body's organs, hormones, and energy systems.

Restoring balance and getting the body back on track can be done through improved diet, cleansing and detoxifying, releasing stress, and getting consistent acupuncture treatments, along with other holistic methods.

394. Do You Have A Tooth or Gum Infection?: Go to your dentist for a thorough cleaning and check-up. A problem with your teeth can weaken the whole body. Do you have any infected teeth? Do you have any cavities that need to be filled? Excessive plaque that needs to be cleaned? Do you need a root canal or a crown? Is there a hidden infection in your teeth that needs to be addressed? It is important that you make sure all infections in your teeth are cleared up and when you begin infertility treatments.

395. Is Your Back or Spine Out of Alignment?: Do not underestimate the role your spine plays in your body's mechanics. There are studies that have shown a link between spinal adjustments and increased fertility, because the nerves to the reproductive system run through the spine. When the back is misaligned, the nerves can misfire and cause a hormone imbalance. Getting your spine and body in alignment can help all your organs function at a higher level and increase your energy flow. Consider an experienced chiropractor and getting an adjustment.

A chiropractor can identify spinal distortions, also called subluxations, that once corrected can improve infertility. If your spine is properly aligned, your nervous system will have a better chance of working at maximum capacity. Think of what happens when your car is properly aligned--your wheels last longer and other parts of your car work better because they are not having to compensate for an unaligned car. The body works in much the same way. If your spine is out of alignment, your legs/hips can also be off and weaken the energy and flow in your lower body. Infections can live in your spine, and if your spine has an infection, it can impact the way your organs communicate with one another.

396. Is Your Body Too Acidic?: When you are trying to get pregnant, one of your goals should be to make the environment within your body as alkaline as possible. Imagine preparing soil for planting—the healthier the soil is, the better chance the seed will have to survive. More than ever before, your body needs to be alkaline, not acidic. Poor eating habits, lack of exercise, and toxic elements in the environment, can cause your body to become acidic. Eating lots of acidic foods result in cervical mucus that is an acidic, which is a hostile environment for sperm. Sperm needs an alkaline environment to survive.

You can test the alkaline/acid in your body with pH strips.

To alkalize your body, start your day by drinking a large glass of water with a freshly squeezed lemon. Foods that alkalize the body include watermelon, apple cider vinegar, artichokes, asparagus, unsalted almonds, coconut oil, lettuce, broccoli, spinach and olive oil.

Foods that help promote an alkaline environment in the body include parsley, garlic, barley grass, green beans, lima beans, zucchini, lemon, beets, asparagus, cabbage, kale, onions, spirulina, flax seeds, sea vegetables, dandelion root, green tea, pumpkin seeds, brussel sprouts. spinach, broccoli, and green leafy vegetables. Figs, apples, grapes, bananas, watermelon, wheatgrass and barley grass are alkaline producing foods. Meat, bread, carbonated drinks, coffee, sugar, fast foods, sodas, muffins, waffles, pancakes, bacon, sausage often promote high levels of yeast and fungi in the body, leading to higher acid levels.

Allergies, arthritis, acne, heart attacks, and weight problems are often linked to an improper pH balance, or acid, in the body.

If your body is alkalized, you are creating an internal environment conducive to pregnancy.

397. Is There Infection In Your Body?: Investigate whether you have any infections in your body. You could have an infection or virus that is weakening you. If so, you may want to consider an antibiotic to get rid of any infections. Juicing and eating lots of garlic can also help fight infections.

398. Do You Have Unknown Allergies?: Are you allergic to corn, wheat or dairy products? Food allergies can sometimes be at the root of infertility problems. Schedule an appointment with an allergist to find out if you have any unknown allergies.

Ask yourself: are there certain foods that make me feel tired, weak, achy, and mildly ill after I eat them? Even if you are not diagnosed as allergic to these foods, stay away from foods that leave you feeling weaker than you felt before you ate them.

399. Do You Have Celiac Disease?: Researchers are finding that women who are allergic to gluten have higher rates of infertility. Even if you are not diagnosed with celiac disease, reducing the gluten you consume can help make your body stronger and more ready to conceive.

400. Is Your Body Cold?: In Chinese medicine, it is believed that the body must be warmed to get pregnant. Avoid iced drinks and very cold foods. Chilled foods cause the body temperature to drop and slows down blood circulation. Do not go barefoot on cold floors. If it is winter and you live in a cold climate, consider wearing warm socks to bed.

Holistic and Alternative Health Treatments To Consider

401. Acupuncture: Without a doubt, acupuncture has been shown to help heal infertility and is one of the best and most effective ways to strengthen your reproductive system. Begin acupuncture treatments as soon as possible. Now! Today! Immediately!

Acupuncture is a wonderful and life changing way to get to the root of some of your fertility problems. Numerous studies have shown that acupuncture dramatically helps infertile couples get pregnant and increases the success rate of IVF and other assisted reproductive technologies.

Acupuncture improves ovarian function, hormonal balance, and helps regulate the chemical pathways in the ovaries, pituitary gland and hypothalamus.

Some studies have shown that acupuncture increases your egg health, and keep eggs healthier than they would normally be without treatment.

Acupuncture also increases blood flow to the ovaries and the uterus, which is very important, because enhanced blood flow can help thicken the lining of the uterus.

Acupuncture also helps correct problems in the endocrine system, which includes the thyroid and hypothalamus, key organs in fertility. Acupuncture can strengthen the liver and kidneys, and help activate the brain to release hormones that stimulate the ovaries, adrenal glands and other organs involved in reproduction.

Acupuncture can moves the body over from a track of disease and dysfunction to a track of health. It enhances your energy, removes energy blocks in the body, and shifts energy back on to proper pathways. If there is a blockage in your energy pathway, acupuncture can clear the blockages and allow energy to flow smoothly. By rerouting blocked energy, acupuncture restores the proper balance of yin and yang in the body.

402. Begin the process of acupuncture and commit to it. To see the benefits of acupuncture takes time and patience. Don't expect to go just once or twice and suddenly have your energy in perfect tune. It takes consistency, but if you stay on track with your weekly treatments, you will eventually see great results.

Try to find someone who has some experience treating infertility patients, but if you can't, that is fine too. If possible, try to go at least twice a week. If you can afford it, go three or four times or as many times as you can.

If money is an issue, you may want to talk with your acupuncturist about getting treatments at a reduced rate. They may be open to giving you a discount if you commit to a certain number of appointments each month, or if you offer to pay up front for five to ten or more appointments at once. Some acupuncturists may discount the treatments for bulk payments. Or some might give you a discount if they know your situation and know you are going to be a long-term customer. In some areas, there are also community acupuncture clinics, also known as group acupuncture, that offer a sliding scale for treatments and are significantly less expensive than one-on-one appointments.

The more acupuncture appointments you can do, the better. Once, during the week I had an IUI scheduled, I went three times to help me conceive, which I ended up doing successfully.

Up until the actual time that you do an IUI or IVF, you can continue acupuncture. There is some disagreement as to whether or not acupuncture should be done once you are pregnant. That is a personal opinion and should be researched and discussed with your acupuncturist. I reserved this wonderful treatment for pre-pregnancy preparation only. If you have an upcoming IVF or IUI, do acupuncture a few times before the procedure.

Bottom line is: you will dramatically increase your chances of if you do acupuncture on a weekly, or preferably, twice weekly basis, for a period of several months.

403. Bio Cleanse : An ionic food bath, also known as a bio cleanse ionic detox foot bath, pulls toxins out of the body through the feet. Positive and negative ions are emitted by the ionic foot bath machine, and helps the body rebalance and eliminate toxins in the kidneys, bowel, liver and skin.

A holistic practitioner in your area may have this machine that can remove yeast, parasites, and heavy metals from your liver, kidneys and muscles. This should only be done as a preparation for infertility treatments, and not once you have started infertility medication or treatments, such as an IUI or IVF. Do not do this if there is any chance you are pregnant. Nor is it safe for anyone with an organ transplant, pacemaker or epilepsy.

404. Lymphatic Massage or Manual Lymphatic Drainage: This is a gentle massage that encourages the natural drainage of the lymph from the tissues in the body. This type of massage is very helpful to your lymph system and is an excellent way to detoxify before an IVF or other types of fertility treatments. Stimulating the lymphatic system helps to drain swollen tissues, enhances the body's immune system, and helps the body's natural waste removal system.

405. Applied Kinesiology: Applied kinesiology can provide you with some incredible emotional healing from trauma or sadness trapped in your body. Our emotions have a physical component and can be energetically trapped in our body, impacting not only our emotional self, but our physical self too. Sometimes, an event or experience can be so painful, that the emotional trauma of it physically lodges itself permanently in the body. This explains why some memories, betrayals, and traumas can feel so recent decades after they occurred, even when we try to let go and forget them.

In applied kinesiology, a chiropractor or holistic practitioner will use what is referred to a "the gun" or activator to release trauma and emotional pain in your body. One way to help release trapped traumas in your body is to write a list of all the people, experiences, and events in your life that have hurt you. Give the kinesiologist this list, and ask them to muscle test and locate where these memories have physicall lodged themselves in your body. Once found, the kinesiologist can activate the "gun" to release or free these emotional energy blocks in your body. Once these traumas leave your body, you'll find yourself feeling better, both emotionally and physically. Your body will no longer be weighed down by intensely negative emotions that do impact your organs and entire body system.

406. Craniosacral therapy: CranioSacral Therapy is a gentle, hands-on form of body work that releases tension in the layer of tissue called the fascia which surrounds the organs and nervous system.

Craniosacral practitioners use light pressure on the skull and lower back to release restrictions on the body's craniosacral system. It is sometimes also done by massage therapists, naturopaths, chiropractors and others who work with the spine, skull and fascia to treat the body's central nervous system. Cranio-sacral can be a powerful tool in releasing past emotional and physical traumas. It can also improve hormone balance and blood flow, and help balance the spinal fluid and nervous system.

407. Blood Type Diet: The body has a chemical reaction to the foods you eat, and some holistic practitioners feel there is some benefit to eating in a way that is compatible with your blood type. If you cannot follow this diet completely, it may help to just be aware of your blood type and take note if you feel more or less energized when you eat foods according to blood type. There are many books available on eating for your blood type.

408. Homeopathy: Homeopathy is a great way to release and unblock emotional traumas or negative patterns that may be affecting your fertility. Homeopathy works on the principle of 'like cures like' and brings the body into balance. Homeopathy uses substances found in nature to give the body the push it needs to begin healing itself.

Homeopathy can be used to treat recurrent miscarriage, irregular ovulation, weakened immune system, and other causes of infertility.

Homeopathy is tailored specifically to each individual's needs according to their symptoms, lifestyle, mental and physical health. Questions like sleep habits, personality, and history will be asked. Treatments are comprised of small doses of what are known as homeopathic remedies.

Common cures include Agnus Castus, also known as Vitex, Sepia 6c for irregular or absent ovulation, Sabin 6c for women who suffer from miscarriages, Phosphorus for treating stress related to infertility and Lycopodium for women who suffer from a dry vagina. The remedies come in tablets, liquid or pellets and are placed under the tongue so they dissolve and are easily absorbed into the system.

409. Ayurvedic Medicine: Ayurvedic medicine is a very ancient holistic healing system developed thousands of years ago in India. In Ayurvedic medicine, it is believed that the root causes of infertility include nervous system imbalances, physical and mental stress, disruption of natural biological rhythms, accumulated toxins in the body, poor nutrition, sluggish digestion and a weakened immune system.

In Ayurvedic medicine, it is believed that a person's physical, spiritual and emotional well-being are all interconnected. Foods considered healing to infertility include grapes, pomegranate, seaweed, almonds, walnuts, mangoes, peaches, plums and pears. Spices recommended are cumin, which purifies the uterus in women and the genitourinary tract in men, turmeric, which improves the interaction between hormones and black cumin. Herbs used to help infertility include raspberry leaves, nettle leaves and flaxseed oil.

Herbs used in Ayurvedic medicine to treat infertility include Ashoka, Shatavari, and Kumari. A fertility-strengthening treatment of a gentle daily warm oil massage of the abdomen in a clockwise motion to support the reproductive organs, followed by a warm bath or shower, is sometimes recommended.

410. Traditional Chinese Medicine: When practitioners of Chinese medicine treat infertility, they work to balance the 'foundation' of the body and the qi, or life energy, that flows through the body, through herbal medicine, acupuncture, massage, dietary therapy and exercise. Emotions, sleeping and eating habits, are all looked at in determining the root cause of infertility. They may treat infertility by suggesting increasing blood flow to the reproductive organs, through acupuncture, massage or exercise. Sometimes they treat infertility by recommending patients avoiding dampness and damp foods such as cheese, butter, alcohol, humid environments and moist basements.

In Chinese medicine, healing one's emotions is key to healing infertility. Two of the most common organs related to fertility are the liver and the lungs. The lungs are related to sadness, grief and holding on, while the liver is connected to frustration, stress, desire and anger.

Calming the mind through acupuncture and saying positive affirmations can help. Being receptive to conception is also important. To do this, think: warm, enveloping, holding, supportive thoughts.

411. Naturopathic Doctors: There are primary care physicians who have also attended naturopathic medical school. They emphasize prevention and self-healing, while focused on identifying the underlying causes of disease. Some of the modalities used in naturopathic medicine to treat infertility include nutrition, homeopathy, hydrotherapy, along with conventional medicine.

412. **Tests You Can Request At the Fertility Clinic:** Don't just wait for your doctor to recommend a test or advanced treatment. Request it! If they won't do it, go somewhere else and find a doctor and/or clinic that will accommodate your requests. Some tests you may want to request include:
- Fibroids or fibroid tumors
-Cysts
-Endometriosis
-Polycystic ovarian syndrome
-Hormone imbalance
-Ovulation problems
-Luteinizing hormone (LH) testing
-Progesterone testing
-Estradiol Level testing
-Hysterosalpingogram
-Laparoscopy to investigate possible scarring, cysts, fibroid tumors or other abnormalities
-Post coital testing
-A thyroid test
-FSH Level

-Fallopian Tube testing, that can include sonohysterogram, hysterosalpingogram, and lapascropy to check if your fallopian tubes are blocked.
-Endometrial biopsy
-Transvaginal ultrasound
-Hysteroscopy: to look for growth or defects in the uterus that cannot be seen with other tests.
- Screen for sexually transmitted diseases

413. **Vitamins and Other Supplements that Can Help Prepare Your Body for Pregnancy:** Start with a high-quality prenatal vitamin and a high-quality mineral supplement. If possible, see a reputable nutritionist or holistic health practitioner to start a balanced vitamin and herb regime.

Remember: some vitamins, herbs and supplements need to be stopped the moment you could be pregnant—some are for pre-pregnancy preparation only, and not safe once you have conceived. Other vitamins and herbs should not be taken at the same time you are taking infertility medications.

414. A High-Quality Pre-Natal Vitamin: It is most important to start taking a pre-natal vitamin before you are pregnant to give your body the nutrients it needs.

415. Omega-3: Some people consider Omega-3 a key part of a fertility health regimen. Omega-3 fats help fertility by regulating hormones, increasing cervical mucus, promoting ovulation and improving the overall quality of the uterus by increasing blood flow to the reproductive organs. Omega-3 supplements also boost the immune system and reduce natural killer cells that can prevent the embryo's implantation in the uterus.

416. Coenzyme 10: This is a supplement both you and your husband should consider taking—and be a supplement that you might consider your new best fertility friend! Recent studies have shown that Co-enzyme Q10 can actually help improve egg quality in older women and improve fertilization rates because it corrects the energy which impacts the division of chromosomes during fertilization.

It can improve the quantity and quality of your eggs, which is key to beating infertility. It is a major cellular antioxidant and can be considered giving your body a high grade fuel to up your cellular energy production process and protect your body from DNA damage. Ubiquinol, the active form of Coenzyme Q10, has demonstrated the ability to improve mitochondrial energy production in aged eggs. Other studies have shown that it also helps improve sperm density and motility in men. This supplement has been shown to improve the rates of conception and live birth in women who are taking it.

417. Folic Acid: You should begin taking folic acid long before you are pregnant in order to build it up in your system. The recommended dosages before pregnancy range from 400 mcg to 600 mcg. When I was trying to conceive, I opted for a higher dose of folic acid.

418. Evening Primrose Oil: This oil is known to help produce fertile quality cervical fluid. This should only be taken BEFORE you are pregnant. STOP taking once if there is even a slight chance you could be pregnant. It aids in conception, but is not be taken at all during pregnancy.

419. Vitamin C: Known as a great friend to fertility, Vitamin C helps improve hormone levels

420. B complex: B6 balances hormone levels and improves low progesterone levels of women affected by luteal phase defect. B12 enhances ovulation and improves the inner lining of the uterus.

421. Vitamin E: Vitamin E an increase cervical mucus in women, prevent egg defects and increase overall egg health. Some studies suggest it can also lengthen the luteal phase of a cycle.

422. Zinc: Helps produce mature eggs ripe for fertilization, maintain proper follicular fluid levels, and regulate hormone levels of estrogen, progesterone and testosterone.

423. Bee Pollen: Stimulates ovarian function, nourishes the ovaries, aids in the production of healthy eggs and normalizes menstrual cycle.

424. Royal Jelly: High in amino acids, proteins and other vitamins. It balances hormones and supports the production of healthy eggs.

425. Calcium: A vital ingredient in triggering growth in embryos. The minerals in calcium help create an alkaline environment in the reproductive tract. It also contains the nutrient that the sperm soaks up and gives help in thrusting towards the egg.

426. Iron: A blood-building nutrient that helps ovulation. Iron deficiency can cause the eggs stored in the ovaries to weaken over time and become unviable. Anemia also makes it impossible for the growing fetus' cells to divide and grow properly.

427. L-Arginine: Known to enhance ovarian response, endometrial receptivity and pregnancy rates. It also increases cervical mucus.

428. **Powerful Foods To Help Cure Your Infertility:** When working towards healing from infertility, never for one moment underestimate the power of the foods you eat. Right now, this moment, you need to begin seeing everything you eat and drink as either a potential healer of your infertility or a potential destroyer of your fertility.

The foods you eat right now could mean the difference between getting pregnant and not getting pregnant. This is how important the food component of your fertility journey is.

 Do not be fooled into thinking that you can drink lots of coffee, eat white flour products, sugar, and processed, fast-foods and it won't impact your body's ability to conceive.

Yes, there are some women who can live off fast food and still get pregnant whenever they choose—but there are also millions of women whose fertility is being stolen by the foods they eat.

To prepare for pregnancy, it is key that you plan, choose and decide to eat as healthy as possible to maximize your body's ability to have a baby. Don't be trapped into thinking that you can eat the way you've always eaten and still heal your body.

If getting pregnant is not coming easily to you, you need to change your eating habits and let go of archaic ideas about food that could be holding your body back.Every time you are tempted by that chocolate bar in the vending machine at work, or a cup of coffee, or a cracker with lots of hydrogenated oil, remind yourself that chocolate bar, or that cup of coffee, or that cracker, could be what ultimately prevents you from having a baby.

If you think a bagel, cream cheese and coffee is a healthy way to start to the day, think again.

It is simple: what you eat can make you weak or make you strong. The right foods can heal your infertility and the wrong ones can rob you of your right to be a mother.

Here are some tips that will help you use food as a way to heal your infertility and prepare your body for pregnancy:

429. Stop Or Reduce Your Coffee Consumption: Do you drink coffee? You need to consider stopping. As much as you can, preferably stop all coffee. If you can't stop, drink no more than a half a cup to a cup a day. That's it. Ideally, do everything you can to say goodbye to coffee for now. Coffee is an enemy of your fertility. Every time you are tempted to drink coffee, remind yourself that this cup of coffee could rob you of the ability to give birth to children. Get rid of all caffeine products in your life. Extreme, maybe, but coffee can weaken key organs, such as the liver, and right now, you need to stack the odds in your favor.

Some studies have shown that women who drink high amounts of coffee take up to three times longer to conceive, and even small amounts of coffee can hamper fertility. To cope with the lack of coffee in your life, you may need to go to bed earlier and eat healthier to compensate for the energy the coffee gave you to get through the day. Coffee cannot be your fuel or main source of energy anymore. Your energy has to come from healthy foods, and other genuinely energy-producing sources. As you detoxify and strengthen your body, your energy will increase and come from your inner core of health—not coffee, an imposter who pretends to hand you energy, but ultimately steals it. Say goodbye to coffee, hello to food sources that genuinely fuel you.

430. Reduce or Eliminate Sugar: Do you eat lots of sweets? Realize that donuts, candy, cake, and other foods with sugar weaken your body and can prevent you from becoming pregnant.

Sugar puts your body in a diseased, acidic state. Sugar can cause hormone imbalances, vitamin deficiencies, high insulin levels, and a compromised immune system. While an occasional sweet is okay, overall you'll want to drastically reduce the sugar in your life.
It can be hard to quit eating all sweets entirely. Many of us have sugar cravings, but overall you want to drastically reduce the amount of sugar you consume.

You'll also need to be be aware and carefully examine the foods you eat that may have hidden sugars in them. Read labels carefully as sugar content varies by brand. Always remember: if its packaged, there is a chance it might have sugar in it.

Foods you need to be aware of for potential sugar content include:

• Yogurt
• Cereals
• Canned vegetables
• Canned soups
• Breakfast bars
• Salad dressing
• Condiments
• White flour products.
• Breads and rolls
• Juices
• Fast foods
• Barbecue sauce
• Soda
• Spaghetti sauce
• Energy drinks
• Dried fruit
• Crackers

Products that list ingredients such as, dextrose, fructose, corn syrup, high-fructose corn syrup, fruit juice concentrate, lactose, sorbitol, xylitol, maltodetrin and turbinado sugar, polydextrose, mannitol, and turbinado sugar. Ingredients ending in 'ose' is often a likely form of sugar.

- Oatmeal
- Protein bars
- Ice tea
- Ketchup
- Frozen meal entrees, even diet ones
- Syrups
- Jelly and jams
- Fruit juice concentrate
- Bouillon cubes
- Bacon
- Luncheon meats

431. Consider Reducing or Eliminating Hydrogenated Oils, Also Known As Trans Fats: Another category of food you need to consider cutting from your diet entirely are foods made with hydrogenated oils, also known as trans fats. Several studies have shown that women with fertility problems eat more trans fats or hydrogenated oils than fertile women. Hydrogenated oil is a man-made food substance used widely throughout the food industry because it lengthens the shelf life of many foods and is cost effective.

Trans fats interfere with the metabolic processes in the body, because they take the place of essential fatty acids that perform critical functions. Trans fats clog up the space that natural fats should occupy, making it difficult for essential nutrients to pass in and out of the cells. Bodily functions are altered by these artificial molecules that enter the system. Various studies have shown that women who eat a diet high in hydrogenated oils are at increased risk for developing endometriosis.

The World Health Organization has tried to outlaw trans fats for decades. Some say trans fats work against the body, because they cause a cell-by-cell failure that destroys the flexibility of healthy cell membranes—basically tearing the body down from the inside out.

Trans fats increase bad cholesterol, block production of chemicals that combat inflammation and benefit the body's hormonal and nervous systems. Trans fats are also linked to heart disease, stroke and diabetes.

They interfere with the absorption of essential fatty acids and DHA, and weaken cell walls and compromise cellular structure.

That means, if you are trying to get pregnant, you need to dramatically reduce eating foods made with hydrogenated oils, corn oil, vegetable oil, transfats and corn syrup.

Be sure to read food labels carefully so you are aware of what products contain hydrogenated oils.

Fast food restaurants often serve a lot of foods loaded with hydrogenated oils. Cake, pancake, biscuit, and cookie mixes are usually made with hydrogenated oils.

Diet foods that promise 'no fat' often have hydrogenated oils.

Labels that say partially hydrogenated, or hydrogenated, contain trans fats. Even foods that promise to be trans fat free may contain up to 0.5 grams of partially hydrogenated oil, a source of trans fats.

Remember that if you see the word 'hydrogenated' or partially hydrogenated, it means it contains a trans fat. Hydrogenated oils are also trans fats, and that includes hydrogenated coconut or soybean oil.

Read labels carefully because hydrogenated oil content can vary by brand.

Begin to replace hydrogenated oils with healthy oils your body needs, such as olive oil, coconut oil and flax seed oil.

It is best to avoid as many pre-packaged foods that you can at this time.

Foods to be aware of can include:

• Commercially baked cakes, cookies, muffins, pies, donuts
• Crackers
• Peanut butter
• Frozen meals
• Frozen bakery items
• French fries
• Whipped toppings
• Margarines
• Shortening
• Cake frosting
• Taco shells
• Microwave popcorn
• Breakfast cereals
• Corn chips and potato chips
• Frozen pizzas and frozen burritos
• Low-fat ice creams
• Pre-made noodle soups and soup mixes
• Bread
• Pasta mixes
• Sauce mixes
• Deep fried foods
• Frozen breakfast foods
• Packaged snacks
• Many different types of candies
• Some salted peanuts
• White bread
• Non-dairy creamers
• Tortillas
• Donuts
• Peanut butter
• Ice cream and low fat ice cream
• Hamburger and hot dog buns
• Movie popcorn
• Frozen pizza
• Refrigerated dough products
• Most fried foods—ask what type of oil the product is fried in
• Piecrust

- Cake mixes
- Pancakes and pancake mixes
- Waffles
- Frozen burgers
- Beef hot dogs
- Refrigerated cookie dough
- Biscuits and sweet rolls
- Refrigerated dough
- Breakfast sandwiches
- Meat sticks
- Crunchy noodles
- Canned chili
- Packaged pudding
- Fish sticks
- Low-fat ice cream
- Frozen burritos
- Noodle soup cups
- Cocoa or hot chocolate mix
- Instant mashed potatoes
- Gravy mixes
- Dips
- Potato chips
- Frozen pot pies
- Sandwiches grilled at a restaurant
- Reduced fat and fat free noodles
- Spreads

432. Consider Eliminating Alcohol: At this time, it is best to stop all alcohol. A glass of wine occasionally when trying to get pregnant might not hurt, but nothing more and no hard liquors. Many studies suggest that the higher your alcohol consumption, the less chance you have of conceiving. Alcohol can impair the detoxifying process that occurs within the liver, and if the liver is working hard to metabolize alcohol, it can become run down and sick. Too much alcohol can also contribute to hormonal imbalances. Alcohol can adversely affect ovulation and affect the body's ability to produce the amino acids necessary for cell development.

433. Cut Down On White Flour Products: How many white flour products do you eat each day? Do you start your day with a bagel, donut or white bread toast? If so, get rid of white flour in your life as much as possible. An occasional bowl of spaghetti may be okay, but in general, you want to reduce the white flour products in your life as much as you can. White flour products, including pasta, bagels and bread, are not health builders and will not advance your goal of becoming pregnant. If you feel extremely weak and lethargic after eating white flour products, you may have celiac disease or a wheat intolerance. Symptoms include stomachaches, fatigue, bloating and flatulence. Check labels and brands. Some sources of white flour can include:

- Alcohol
- Crackers
- Cereals
- Corn flour
- Cake and cookie mixes
- Pancake mixes
- Muffin mixes
- Puddings
- Pretzels
- Donuts
- Foods with artificial colorings and preservatives
- Sweet and sour glazes
- Sweet sauces
- Soy sauce
- Ice cream cones
- Foods containing malt
- Powdered or canned soups
- Fast foods
- Gravies

Instead, choose wheat-free products made from rice, oat, rye, and puffed rice cereals.

434. Reduce Your Intake Of Diet Foods or Foods with Sugar Substitutes: You may want to consider reducing your intake of diet foods, diet drinks or foods with sugar substitutes or artificial sweeteners. Some experts on fertility recommend avoiding sweeteners listed on labels as aspartame, sucralose, acesulfame potassium, also listed as acesulfame k and ACE, neotame, and saccharin.

Consider cutting back or eliminating diet drinks and powdered drinks that contain any of these sweeteners. These sweeteners may also be in some chewing gums and ice creams.

Some doctors have concluded that these artificial sweeteners interfere with fetal development, and act as 'instant birth control.' Aspartame is considered a endocrine disrupting chemical, by some medical providers.

Artificial sweeteners and sugar substitutes negatively impact the hormones in the pituitary glands, thyroid and ovaries.

Hidden sources of these artificial sweeteners can include:

- Breads
- Jello
- Gelatins
- Toothpaste
- Breath mints
- Drink mixes
- Syrups
- Jellies
- Cereals
- Sugar-free candies

435. Reduce or Eliminate Soy: Some studies suggest that high levels of soy act as endocrine disrupters and decrease fertility. The phytoestrogens found in soy interfere with endocrine function and can mimic the female hormone oestrogen, which disrupts the normal production of sex hormones. Soy can decrease the follicle-stimulating hormone (FSH), as well as the leutinizing hormone.

Many soy products are genetically engineered and can reduce the body's ability to absorb minerals. Some soy isoflavones mimic estrogen—which means the body thinks it has estrogen it doesn't have, thus causing hormone imbalances. Some studies have also shown that soy can lead to thyroid problems, such as hypothyroidism.

Soy derivatives are often labeled under different names, including mono-diglyceride, soya, soja, yuba, TSF or textured soy flour, TSP textured soy protein, TVP textured vegetable protein, lecithin, and MSG, yeast extract, soy protein.

Hidden sources of soy include:

• Protein bars
• Meal replacement shakes
• Bottled fruit drinks
• Soups
• Sauces
• Baked goods
• Breakfast cereals
• Chewing gum
• Chocolate
• Bread
• Microwave meals
• Frozen pizzas
• Processed meat
• Soy milk
• Soy beans
• Corn chips
• Canned tuna

436. Avoid Fish Known To Potentially Have High Mercury Levels: Due to high mercury levels, some types of fish are best avoided or eaten rarely when trying to get pregnant. These include swordfish, shark, grouper, marlin, orange roughy, tilefish, mackerel, tuna, bluefish, lobster, halibut, croaker and bass saltwater. The fish with the reported lowest amounts of mercury include calamari, crab, pollock, scallops, salmon, shrimp, clams, and others, but these also need to be eaten in moderation.

437. No MSG: Avoid foods that could have monosodium glutamate, also known as MSG. Foods that might contain MSG include potato chips, Chinese food, meat seasonings and packaged soups. MSG can appear on labels as autolyzed yeast, maltodextrin, hydrolyzed pea protein.

438. Other Foods To Avoid:

• Avoid raw or undercooked meats.
• Avoid raw or undercooked eggs.
• Stay Away From Fast Food
• Avoid Deli Meats

Fertility-Strengthening Foods

439. Eat More Vegetables: Here's a simple fact that will increase your fertility: the more vegetables you eat, the more fertile you will be.

Repeat: More vegetables you eat, the healthier and more fertile you will be. Implant that thought in your brain, please, please, please.

Your diet should include a lot of vegetables every single day.

Note the word: a lot.

In fact, most of the foods you eat, starting with breakfast, should be vegetables.

Starting now, the way you eat should revolve around vegetables.

Vegetables should no longer be just a small side dish you include with dinner—they should be the main course, present at almost every meal and every snack you eat. They are the key to healing your body. You need to start looking at vegetables in a way that is not traditional in our culture—as your main source of food.

Vegetables should become part of your breakfast, your snacks, lunch and dinner. You want to find as many ways as you can to dramatically increase the vegetables you eat daily.

For lunch, eat a big bowl of romaine lettuce. Munch on parsley for a snack. Roast some asparagus and olive oil to eat before bed. Bake some sweet potatoes and olive oil for snack. Include spinach in your salads or sandwiches.

Slice up some peppers, carrots, red and green peppers, tomatoes, and seaweeds and place in bags so you have easy-to-eat snacks ready throughout the day.

Don't allow a busy schedule to force you to have to run to the nearest fast food drive-through because you are starving and need to just fill your stomach. At night before bed, prepare a salad of chicory and romaine lettuce. Or just wash some kale or spinach, put in a bag, and have it on your way home from work.

Nibble on broccoli before bed. Include a salad with every meal. Put vegetables on your pizza, in your tomato sauces, soups and stews.

Instead of a sandwich of deli meat, how about a sandwich of tomato and basil, broccoli and cheese, or spinach and tomato?

Eat vegetables the way you would eat fruit—a whole cucumber, a whole tomato, a whole carrot.

Select one or two days a week and eat only vegetables the entire day. Start your day with a green veggie drink or smoothie, add some flaxseed, coconut oil, maca, honey and spirulina.

Make a vegetable breakfast wrap, top an multi-grain English muffin with onions, peppers, and tomatoes. Create dips with vegetables—and then dip your vegetables! Add vegetables to spreads like hummus or mashed avocados. Make vegetable submarine sandwiches, with healthy bread and lots of olive oil.

Juicing or smoothies are a great way to include more vegetables in your diet. Drink a glass of spinach juice each day. Juice parsley, kale, beets, and garlic once or twice a day.

Start including garlic in many of your recipes as you can. Chew on garlic, juice garlic and make garlic part of your daily eating routine.

Remember: from now on, vegetables should make up more than 60 to 70 percent of the foods you eat each day.

Some super fertility vegetables include:

• Spinach is high in iron and folic acid, two important nutrients for reproductive health. Women with low iron intakes are at greater risk for ovulatory fertility.

To enhance absorption of iron from spinach, combine it with a food that contains vitamin C, such as broccoli, strawberries, green peppers or oranges.

• Alfalfa provides the body with a rich source of essential minerals important for reproductive health.

• Broccoli and cabbage contain a phytonutrient that helps with estrogen metabolism.

• Yams and sweet potatoes contain a compound called diosgenins which impacts hormonal patterns and increases ovulation. Yams have massive amounts of vitamin A that improve cervical fluid and follicle development. They are also loaded with beta carotene that helps regulate the menstrual cycle. It also has high amounts of Vitamin B which helps regulate hormones. They also help stabilize blood sugar— and the more stable your sugar levels, the better your ovulation will be.

• Asparagus is also a high fertility food.

• Wheat Grass is one of the best sources of living chlorophyll. It helps balance the PH levels in the body and is high in magnesium, which helps restore sex hormones.

• Spirulina is a great source of the essential acid GLA.

• Chlorella: a green algae that helps the body cleanse and detoxify.

Here is a checklist to help you keep track of the vegetables you eat each day:

Vegetables to eat every day include:

--Spinach
--Yams and Sweet Potatoes
--Peppers
--Broccoli
--Arugula
--Asparagus
--Romaine
--Seaweed
--Garlic
--Cabbage
--Dandelion greens
--Romaine Lettuce
--Red Peppers
--Dark green lettuce
--Kale
--Asparagus
--Beets
--Seaweeds
--Brussel sprouts

440. Eat More Fruits: Along with eating as many vegetables as possible, start including more fruits in your diet. Fruits are packed with antioxidants, which protect the body from cell aging and damage—including cells in the reproductive system, like your eggs.

Start eating one or two bowls of blueberries for breakfast. Blueberries have phytonutrients that have hormone balancing properties that impact ovulation.

Many holistic practitioners recommend eating avocados to boost fertility, because they are a great source of Vitamin E, a huge fertility booster. Avocados help regulate both ovulation and production of cervical mucus. They are rich in folic acid and vitamin B6, which helps prevent luteal phase defect.

Bananas are full of potassium, Vitamin C and fiber, and bromelain which increases sex hormone production.

Slice up some papaya as your bedtime snack, have two or three bowls of strawberries, blackberries, raspberries and blueberries for breakfast, bring apples to work.

Eat fresh pineapple daily, including the pineapple core. Pineapple contains bromelain that aids in implantation. Pineapple is also one the best natural sources of manganese, an important mineral that triggers production of various reproductive hormones. Low levels of this mineral have been reported to be associated with difficulty conceiving. Note: if you are already taking aspirin, be aware that pineapple might thin your blood.

Pomegranates are considered a fertility super food.

Eat lots of fruits that contain Vitamin C, such as oranges, kiwi, blueberries and strawberries, a nutrient key to fertile health.

Fruits to include in your daily diet:

-Plums
-Blueberries
-Strawberries
-Bananas
-Grapes
-Cantaloupe
-Oranges
-Apples
-Mangoes
-Bananas
-Blueberries

-Lemons
-Pomegranate
-Figs
-Apricots
-Prunes
-Peaches
-Blackberries

441. Eat More Beans: Beans are an essential food for developing good follicle quality. Black beans are considered by some to be a reproductive tonic. Lentils are also a healthy source of iron that support ovulation and aid fertility. Aduki beans are considered to support the Kidney Qi, which is essential for reproductive function.

442. Eat More Nuts: Start including lots of nuts in your diet, such as walnuts, almonds, and brazil nuts. Nuts have high amounts of Omega 3 and Omega 6, which have been known to improve sperm quality and egg quality.

Nuts can enhance pancreas function, thus helping to regulate insulin and blood sugar levels in the body. Almonds contain L-arginine and zinc which are important nutrients to the reproductive system.
Walnuts are high in protein and folic acid and are an excellent source of omega-3 fatty acids. Almonds contain high levels of zinc and L-arginine, which are important nutrients to the reproductive system.

443. Eat More Seeds: Seeds contain a lot of omega 3s which are key to fertility. Pumpkin seeds which contain zinc, an important nutrient in egg production. Sunflower seeds and sesame seeds provide healthy fats. Black sesame seeds can help enhance liver function and sesame seeds are rich in minerals.

444. Healthy Oils: Because fat intake is so vital to fertility, include olive oil, coconut oil and flaxseed oil in your diet. Healthy fats, as opposed to trans fats, can make the body more fertile, reduce inflammation in the body and increase insulin sensitivity. Olive oil, like avocados, has monounsaturated fat, which helps assist in reproduction. Some people have taken a mixture of olive oil, honey and mustard seed to enhance their fertility.

Flax seed oil helps the hormones hit the receptor cells in a precise way so they can work at their maximum capacity. This helps the membranes in the receptor cells be more flexible, run more smoothly and makes it easier for hormones to bind with. It also encourages healing in the uterus, and is rich in omega fatty acids.

Coconut oil helps maintain hormonal balance for reproduction and helps thyroid function and ovulation cycles.

445. Honey: Bee pollen stimulates ovarian function. It is also rich in minerals such as copper, potassium, and zinc and also has 20 of the 22 known amino acids. Bee pollen contains natural hormonal substances that stimulate and nourish the reproductive system, stimulate ovarian function and increase the health and biological value of the egg.

446. Wild Salmon: According to Chinese medicine, salmon is good for nourishing the yin and blood, helping to generate healthy follicles and ample amounts of cervical fluid.

447. Lean Cuts of Meat: When possible, choose lean cuts of meat. An overload of heavy red meat can work against your fertility.

448. Drink Lots of Good Quality Water: Drinking a lot of the right water can do so much to enhance your fertility. Water increases cervical fluid which is key in conception. Water can help sperm stay alive for days. Water also facilitates the transport of hormones and plumps up follicles.

The key is that along with drinking a lot of water, you need to drink high-quality water. Do you drink tap water? What is the quality of the water in your community? For now, start buying purified water and use it for all your drinking and cooking needs. Put a filter on your tap water. As much as you can, stop drinking water out of plastic bottles that can contain the chemical bisphenol A, also known as BPA. Keep your water stored in glass containers, rather than plastic.

449. Start Your Day Drinking Lemon in Warm Water: Lemon enhances your immunity and increases liver and digestive health.

150. Brown Rice: Replace white rice with brown rice for enhanced nutrition. Brown rice is a slow carbohydrate, which means a gradual rise in blood sugar after being eaten.

451. Green Tea: For better quality eggs and more viable embryos, consider drinking two or more cups of green tea a day. Green tea contains polyphenols and hypoxanthine, which increase the percentage of viable embryos. Hypoxanthine enhances the follicular fluid that helps eggs mature and be ready for fertilization.

Green tea also contains polyhenols that act as an antioxidant and gets rid of unwanted toxins in the body. Green tea can help repair oxidative damage that occurs in the body due to stress, aging and the environment. Drink in moderation, as it can decrease the body's absorption of iron and decrease the effects of folic acid, so you might want to make sure you taking adequate amounts of iron and folic acid at the same time.

You should reduce the amount of green tea you drink once you are pregnant or if there is even a slight chance you are pregnant. The polyphenols in green tea that help prevent chromosomal abnormalities in your eggs can cause an embryo to miscarry or fail to implant.

452. Pomegranates and Natural Pomegranate Juice: Pomegranates help boost fertility by increasing blood flow to the uterus and thickening the uterine lining. They also help balance the hormones estrogen and progesterone. The antioxidants in pomegranates help prevent DNA damage to eggs and contain folic acid, essential during the early stages of a pregnancy.

453. Pineapple Core: Cut the core into round sections and eat after embryo transfers to help implantation. The bromelain found in the core reduces inflammation and improves uterine lining.

454. Brewer's Yeast: Brewer's yeast is a great source of B complex, and is rich in minerals like zinc, iron and chromium.

Here are some more ways to maximize your fertility and improve your chances of conceiving:

455. Try Robitussin: Some women swear by Robitussin (guaifenesin) cough syrup because it is believed to help thin cervical fluid.

456. Baby Aspirin: Ask your doctor if baby aspirin might be something you should consider. Some research has shown that low doses of aspirin can help increase blood flow to the uterine lining and can enhance ovarian response. Some studies have also shown it reduces the risk of miscarriage.

457. You may have heard that when you are trying to get pregnant, intercourse should only take place every few days to help build sperm levels. This is actually untrue. The more you do it, the better – so when you are ovulating, enjoy every moment you have together!

458. Do not use any lubricants or oils when trying to get pregnant.

459. Find intimate positions that allow for deep penetration.

460. After intercourse, remain in bed for 30 minutes.

461. Do not urinate 30 minutes after intercourse.

462. Go to acupuncture once or twice a few days before an IUI or IVF to balance and strengthen your body.

463. If you are already seeing a myofascial release specialist or a kinesiologist, get a treatment a few days before your IUI or IVF to help prepare your body to receive.

How to increase your chances of conceiving before and after your IUI or IVF.

464. Can you spend a few days at a local beach or lake right after an IVF? Spending time in sunlight also helps.

465. Eat extra healthy foods the week of the IUI and IVF, and, of course, afterwards.

466. After an IUI, ask if you can remain on the table for 25 to 40 minutes. Put your legs up against the wall to help the sperm travel to your eggs. Or don't ask permission if you think the answer is going to be no—and just take a really, really long time dressing. They can't force you out.

467. Some studies suggest that touching, caressing and other forms of physical stimulation can increase hormones, thus improving chances for conception. Before an IUI or IVF, make out with your husband, touch each another, and get yourself a little bit 'in the mood.'

468. Do not urinate 30 minutes after an IUI or IVF.

469. **Getting Your Guy Ready: The Ultimate Male Fertility Preparation Program**: Along with getting yourself prepared for pregnancy, it is important to help your husband and/or partner become as fertile as possible. Don't panic if your guy was diagnosed with a low sperm count. Just as there are many things a woman can do to maximize her fertility, there are also many things a man can do to improve the quality, quantity, and speed of his sperm.

Whether or not your guy was diagnosed with any specific problem, it is important to address his fertility because underlying, undiagnosed problems could exist that are not being caught.

Some causes of inadequate sperm production include hormone imbalances, post-testicular issues with plumping or ejaculation, trauma or accidents, varicocele, or dilated veins in the scrotum, undescended testis/testes, excessive xenoestrogen, which are environmental estrogen exposure; infectious disease of the epidydimis, a diseased endocrine (glandular) system affecting the hypothalamus, pituitary, thyroid, adrenals and the testes, resulting in low DHEA and testosterone levels, congenital abnormalities, urethral stricture, malnutrition, especially protein deficiency. It can sometimes take two to three months to improve the quality of sperm, so you'll want to begin preparing as soon as possible.

470. Here are some of the tests your husband/partner can request:

• Sperm analysis, including a sperm antibody test, which can determine sperm count, motility, morphology (shape), seminal fluid, volume of ejaculation, and pH level.

• A Hormone Analysis: Hormones include testosterone, follicle stimulating hormone, and lutinizeing hormone which are critical to sperm production. You may also want to have analyzed prolacin levels, thyroid stimulating hormone, sand ex-hormone binding globulin.

• Scrotal Doppler Ultrasound: measures the size of the testicle and look for blockages that involve transport of sperm out of the testicle.

• Transrectal Ultrasound: ultrasound technology is used to image the reproductive tract.

• A blood test to check for infections and hormone levels.

• A white blood cell count to detect infection, past infection, inflammation, low levels of inhibin B, or the compound alpha-glucosidase.

• Forward progression: this test measures the amount of forward movement in the sperm.

• Kruger morphology: if an abnormal morphology is found, this test allows the specialists to examine the sperm structure in great detail.

• Anti-sperm antibodies: this means the male has created an immunological response toward the sperm cells

• Sperm agglutination: sperm is examined to see whether there is any clumping together of the cells. Sperm agglutination can indicate the presence of sperm antibodies or bacterial infection.

• Viability: this test is performed if the sperm analysis shows that less than 30 percent of the sperm are motile. This test determines whether or not there is a presence of live sperm.

• Fructose: this test determines whether there is a blockage or no sperm at all being produced.

• An often overlooked cause of infertility in men is low-grade infection in the male urinary tract. Symptoms are often subtle and hard to diagnose, but they can include chills, fever, increased urination and intense burning during urination. Some physicians recommend culturing a semen sample to detect this mild infection.

Here are some cleanses for men to consider before beginning infertility treatments:

470. A Parasite Cleanse: Parasites can weaken sperm on a very hard-to-detect level. Health food stores carry 30-day parasite cleanses that can effectively remove parasites from the body.

471. Heavy Metal Cleanse: Chemicals, pesticides and toxins in our environment have greatly impacted male fertility. Many men suffer from low-quality sperm because of these environmental toxins and chemicals. If possible, consider a heavy metal cleanse that can help remove these chemicals.

472. Liver Cleanse: Just as detoxifying the liver is key to healing female infertility, it is equally important for men. Consider having your partner do a liver cleanse. The liver helps to filter toxins from the body, including excess hormones.

473. Candida-Yeast Cleanse: can help rid the body of toxins.

474. Colon Hydrotherapy: A colon cleanse can eradicate years of toxins in the large intestine, reducing the burden on the liver, pancreas, gall bladder and kidney.

Holistic and Alternative Health Treatments to Consider:

475. Acupuncture: Acupuncture has been known to help men who have a low sperm count. It may be helpful for your partner to begin weekly or twice-weekly acupuncture treatments.

Make sure to let the acupuncturist know that you are looking to strengthen your husband's sperm Acupuncture points can help redirect Qi (energy) to key points in the body that assist in the smooth flow of blood to the penis and scrotum.

Vitamins and Supplements That Often Help Male Infertility:

476. Vitamin C: High-quality vitamin C supplements enhance sperm development. Some recommend 2,000 to 6,000 milligrams daily to prevent sperm from clumping or sticking together. Foods that contain lots of Vitamin C include strawberries, citrus fruits, cherries, cantaloupe, broccoli, tomatoes, sweet peppers, mangos, kiwi, pineapple, grapes, peas, potatoes, parsley and spinach. Keep a bowl of these foods washed and easily available.

477. Zinc: is very important to sperm quality because it increases testosterone levels, sperm count and sperm motility. Men should consider taking a zinc supplement or a high-quality multivitamin that contains zinc, as a zinc deficiency has been shown to cause or reduce male infertility. In addition to taking a supplement, foods high in zinc include oysters, organic meats, lean beef, turkey, lamb, herring, wheat germ, beans, sunflower and pumpkin seeds.

478. L-Arginine: is an amino acid that enhances low sperm counts and poor motility. It is found in high amounts in the head of the sperm. Studies show that sperm and semen volume double with this amino acid. Food sources of L-arginine include nuts, raisins, sesame seeds, brown rice, peanuts, almonds chocolate, meat and poultry.

479. A Multivitamin: taken daily.

480. Vitamin E: Studies have shown that Vitamin E increases sperm health and motility.

481. Folic acid: Studies suggest that men with low levels of this key B vitamin have trouble producing healthy sperm. Folic acid reportedly improves sperm motility and sperm structure. Food sources include leafy greens, orange juice and spinach.

482. Korean Ginseng: enhances testosterone and sperm levels.

483. Selenium: should be taken as part of a quality multi-vitamin.

484. Coenzyme Q10: increases energy production in the sperm and can increase motility and quality of sperm.

485. Omega-3: acts as a hormone regulator.

486. Vitamin A: helps enhance male hormones.

487. B-complex: This vitamin is very important to male fertility. Vitamin B6 and B12 have been reported to improve sperm counts. Vitamin B12 can increase the quantity and quality of your guy's sperm. Foods that contain B vitamins include lamb, sardines and salmon.

488. Calcium-Magnesium: aids Vitamin B absorption.

489. Vitamin A: increases male hormones. Eat plenty of vegetables, fruit, oily fish and dark green leafy vegetables.

490. Royal Jelly: can help optimize hormonal balance.

491. Manganese deficiency: is known to result in testicular degeneration. Foods with manganese include: whole grains, green vegetables, carrots, broccoli, beans, nuts, pineapples, oats, rye and eggs.

More Things Your Guy Can Do To Improve His Fertility:

492. Visit The Dentist: Make sure your husband has his teeth cleaned, thus eliminating the possibility of infections in the gums or teeth.

493. Consider His Weight: Too much or too little body fat can disrupt production of reproductive hormones, thus reducing sperm count. Try to help your husband/partner lose weight, especially scrotal fat, which can act like a warm blanket over the scrotum and elevate sperm temperatures, which in turn, kill and immobilize sperm. Excess fat around the waist is often associated with decreased male fertility.

494. Reduce Stress: Encourage your husband/partner to take steps to reduce stress, as stress has been shown to negatively impact male reproductive hormones and lower testosterone.

495. Drink Lots of Water: Make sure your partner is drinking plenty of high-quality, filtered water each day.

496. Touch, Touch and Touch Some More: Stimulation increases hormones and improves fertility. Touch each other at length before intercourse to increase hormones, both his and yours.

497. Ejaculate Often: Sex is good for sperm, because the less time spent in storage, the higher quality it will be and less DNA damage.

498. Enjoy More Sunshine: Encourage your guy to get outside 10 to 15 minutes a day.

499. Balance The Body's Flora: Eating a diet rich in nuts, seeds, fruits and vegetables can help encourage healthy sperm. Limit sugar, processed foods and encourage your guy to take a probiotic to improve digestive health and reduce inflammation. Reducing the amount of gluten consumed is also important. Restore the acid-alkaline balance in the reproductive system to the proper sperm pH. A diet high in acid-producing foods such as meat, white flour, sugar, alcohol, coffee and soft drinks is to be avoided. Low sperm count or morphology is often caused by hormonal imbalance, and an over-stressed endocrine system.

What Your Guy Should Avoid To Protect His Fertility:

500. Keep It Loose: Have your partner wear loose fitting boxer shorts, instead of tight underwear. Avoid boxers, briefs or bikinis. No tight clothes around the genitals please.

501. Just Say No To Lubricants: Avoid lubricants during sex. Lotions or lubricants can interfere with sperm motility.

502. Don't Let His Sperm Get Too Hot: Heat can deter the healthy development of sperm. Genitals should be kept cool when possible. Lap top computers can increase scrotal temperature, which hurts sperm production.

503. Avoid hot tubs, saunas and Jacuzzis. Wear cotton boxer shorts rather than jockey shorts to keep sperm from overheating. Avoid long drives, and never let him put his cell phone in between his legs while driving. Avoid hot baths or overly long hot showers.

504. If your guy has a job that requires him to sit a lot each day, this could be causing high testicle heat. Encourage him to get up and walk every few hours.

505. Avoid heated car seats, electric blankets and heating pads that increase testicular temperatures—always remember sperm works better when it is cool!

506. If there is a chance that your partner is experiencing too much heat in his genital area, you may want to try artificially cooling his testicles with ice, a cold bath or shower. Always remember: Sperm counts are higher in the cold weather and in the morning.

507. Stop All Cigarette Smoking: Smoking reduces sperm count and motility. It also increases the risk of genetic defects in an embryo. All smoking should be stopped.

508. No Marijuana: Chemicals from marijuana have been reported to build up in the testicles and can cause impotence and a lower sperm count.

509. Take A Look At Prescription Drugs: If your husband is on medication, you may want to evaluate if it is safe for him to take a break while you are trying to conceive. Some prescription drugs can negatively effect sperm count. This is a matter to be decided with a doctor's approval and notification, as some medications are absolutely necessary for various mental and physical health conditions.

510. Reduce Bicycling Activity: Bicycling can raise scrotal temperature and critical arteries and nerves can be damaged by repeatedly banging the groin against the seat.

511. No Oral Sex: Saliva can kill sperm. Avoid oral sex at this time.

512. No Extreme Exercise: Extreme exercise can lower the sperm count.

513. Cut Down Or Reduce Alcohol: Alcohol interferes with the secretion of testosterone and lowers sperm count. Alcohol can also depletes vitamins and minerals in the body and an overworked liver can cause a rise in estrogen

514. Stay Away From Water Bottles That Contain Bisphenol A (BPA): Be aware of Bisphenol A (known as BPA) a hormone-disrupting chemical that is a common ingredient in water bottles, canned goods, and other products. Researchers have found that men with higher urine levels of BPA have decreased sperm concentration, decreased total sperm count, decreased sperm vitality and decreased sperm motility. BPA can also be found on cash register receipts and metal cans.

515. Avoid Soaps and Deodorants That Contain Phthalates: Phthalates are another group of chemicals that have been shown to wreak havoc with reproductive health. They are commonly found in vinyl flooring, detergents, soap, shampoo, deodorants, fragrances, hair spray, plastic bags, vinyl shower curtains, scented soaps, cleaners, garden hoses, and sex toys.

516. Be Aware of Chemicals In His Environment: Other chemicals that are linked to decreased fertility include: Methoxychlor and Vinclozin, an insectide and fungicide, non-fermented soy products that contain hormone-like substances, and fluoride.

Avoid plastic containers for food storage, plastic bottles, wraps and utensils. Be aware of office paper products whitened with chlorine. Use only non-bleached coffee filters, paper, napkins and toilet tissue to reduce dioxin exposure.

517. No Chlorine Products: Avoid chlorinated tap water, chlorine bleach and other chlorinated products.

518. No Deodorants: Avoid synthetic deodorants and use only organic products whenever possible.

519. Reduce Cell Phone Usage and Contact: Cell phones can negatively impact the brain's pituitary output. Ask your guy to cut down on using his phone, and tell him not to carry it in his pocket. Try to encourage him to keep wireless items that transmit EMFs away from his body.

520. Reduce WIFI Usage: Wifi signals contain EMFs that have been found to lower sperm count.

521. No anabolic steroids

522. Some studies suggest anti-ulcer drugs decrease sperm count

523. Avoid Cottonseed toxins hidden in food

524. Avoid pesticides

525. Avoid growth hormones

526. Reduce or Eliminate If Possible Caffeine: Excessive amounts of caffine can impact sperm counts. Caffeine, found in tea, coffee, chocolate, cola, energy drinks, some medications, and stimulants to keep people awake, should be reduced or eliminated.

527. Reduce Contact With Lawn Care Products: Stop using bug sprays, lawn sprays or pesticides to treat lawn and garden.

528. No More Microwaves: Do not microwave food in plastic.

529. No Polyester: Stop wearing polyester clothes.

Fertility-Enhancing Foods for Men

Here are the foods your guy should eat to maximize his fertility.

530. Lots of Green Vegetables: Green vegetables are needed to make your guy's body more alkaline. Juicing a glass of green juice each day is one way to ensure your husband has the greens he needs.

531. Spinach is high in potassium, which improves sperm concentration.

532. Cauliflower provides choline, that has been shown to improve sperm quality.

533. Add extra tomatoes to his salad, as some studies have shown that the lycopene in tomatoes increase sperm count.

534. Red peppers, kiwi, lemons and strawberries are all high in Vitamin C which has been shown to improve sperm count and motility.

535. Sardines are rich in Omega 3's and a good source of Coenzyme Q10.

536. Avocado has L-carnitine which promotes healthy sperm, can boost sperm motility and is packed with Vitamin E, Vitamin B6 and folic acid.

537. Pumpkin seeds are high in zinc, loaded with omega-3 and should be a daily part of his diet.

538. Broccoli is high in selenium

539. Wheat germ and almonds are high in Vitamin E

540. Whole grains like oatmeal and brown rice

541. Extra-virgin olive oil

542. Oysters contain a high level of zinc, which helps increase production of sperm and testosterone.

543. Brazil nuts are rich in selenium, a mineral that boosts sperm production and mobility.

544. Walnuts contains arginine, which increases semen volume and Omega-3s that improve blood flow to the penis.

545. Molasses

546. Apricots

547. Watermelon

548. Sesame seeds

549. Maca

550. Spirulina

551. Foods High In Antioxidants: Sperm is damaged by free radicals and antioxidants can prevent cell damage. High antioxidant foods include: blueberries, blackberries, kale, garlic, Brussels sprouts, plums, red peppers, broccoli and red peppers.

552. Asparagus: contain high amounts of Vitamin C, which prevents sperm from oxidizing and protects the cells of testes.

553. Bananas: contain bromelain, that help increase stamina and boosts the body's ability to make sperm.

554. Wild fish

555. Dark chocolate contains L-Arginine, an amino acid related to the arginine in walnuts.

556. Garlic contains allicin which increases blood flow to the genitals.

557. Pomegranate contains an intense cocktail of antioxidants that can lower a chemical in the blood called malondialidehyde that destroys sperm.

558. Organic Free Range Meat: Some nutritionists recommend eating organically-raised, free range meats, instead of conventional meat that contains hormones and antibiotics. Eat grass fed and organic cattle.

Conventionally raised cattle can sometimes contain high levels of hormones and antibiotics which can contribute to estrogen dominate conditions.

559. Free Range Organic Chicken: Conventionally raised chicken is sometimes full of antibiotics and hormones which can negatively impact hormonal health.

560. Kiwi fruit is high in zinc, which helps protect sperm from chromosomal and bacterial damage.

Foods To Avoid or Eliminate:

561. Your partner should eliminate, or at least cut down, on alcohol, beer and wine while you are trying to get pregnant. Alcohol can lower sperm count, weaken sperm, and impede the secretion of testosterone. Studies have shown that alcohol can decrease sperm count for as much as three months after a big drinking fest.

562. Encourage your partner to avoid sugar. Eating lots of sugar often results in hormone imbalances and robs the body of key nutrients.

563. Cut down or avoid whenever possible white flour or gluten. If someone is sensitive to gluten, it can cause malabsorption of important nutrients, such as zinc, and increase inflammation throughout the body.

564. Reduce or avoid foods with hydrogenated oil as much as possible.

565. Reduce or avoid caffeine, which can reduce sperm count and motility. Caffeine is also detrimental to adrenal function, a gland key in productive hormones. The constant stress of caffeine can cause the body to focus on dealing with stress hormones, instead of reproductive hormones.

566. Reduce or avoid animal products with a high fat content that contain hormones.

567. No fried foods

568. No hot sauce

569. Avoid fried, charcoal-broiled or barbecued forms of cooking.

570. Avoid soy. Soy is high in phyto estrogens, which can upset the hormonal balance in man. The estrogen-like compounds in soy can dramatically lower sperm counts. Texturized soy protein is in many meat substances used in fast food chains, and is also found in cereal, snack crackers and protein shakes.

571. Avoid soda

572. Stop drinking milk for now, since many dairy cows are fed estrogens to produce more milk. If you must drink milk, try to drink milk that is organic and not from estrogen-fed cows. Dairy that is not organic may contain hormones and antibiotics which can contribute to increased estrogen levels in the body. Keep dairy to a minimum.

573. Avoid processed grains, GMO corn and corn products, and corn chips.

Conditions To Have Checked

574. Be sure your husband is aware of any food allergies he may have.

575. Some cases of male infertility are linked to viruses. It would be helpful for your partner to do a parasite cleanse. Investigate whether your guy has an infection, which could be lowering his sperm count.

576. Micro-organisms and bacteria may be the cause of fertility problems. Approximately 15% of cases of male factor infertility are reportedly caused by bacteria, parasites or viruses.

577. Chlamydia

578. Elevated prolactin levels

579. Triglycerides: a sign of metabolic syndrome and insulin resistance

More tips for your guy:

580. There is some research that suggests that sperm levels are highest in the morning, and this could be something to speak to your doctor about when scheduling IVFs and IUI's.

How To Prepare For the Journey Through Infertility

581. Prepare To Take Responsibility for Your Own Healing: This journey is your responsibility and yours alone. Your journey to motherhood is not the responsibility of your doctor, your husband, your mother, or your best friend.

You will ultimately fare better if you take responsibility for your infertility treatments, rather than hoping someone is going to come and pave the way for you or rescue you.

You are in charge and responsible for all the hard work your infertility treatments will demand and require.

Accepting the responsibility of finding a good doctor, showing up to all your appointments, and doing whatever it takes to heal your body, will empower you to make good choices, be organized, self-disciplined, and do whatever you can to improve your chances of conceiving the baby you so deserve. You are the one that must go to the appointments, take the medications, change whatever needs to be changed and sacrifice whatever needs to be sacrificed, in the quest to have a baby. You are in charge. You make the choices. You ask the questions.

You do the research. You explore your options. You ask to try another medication. You change doctors. You eat healthy. You show up on time for the appointments. The choices, the actions, are all up to you.

You want this baby, you need to understand you are the driver.

You are not a child resting easily in the arms of your doctor or anyone else.

Relying on the word of any one doctor, or any one clinic, or any one person, is a big mistake. Starting right now, you need to take responsibility for your treatment--not hand it over to anyone or rely totally on anyone else.

 Many women have made the mistake of letting the course of their treatment be dictated by one person--usually a medical professional--only to find out later that person had been on the wrong track.

By putting yourself firmly in the driver's seat, you will not be afraid to ask for things, push for more, change course when you see the need. You will not be tethered to a treatment that is not working for you. Nor will you be a victim to whatever some authority figure sees fit for you, especially if their pronouncement or decision isn't bringing you the desired results.

Stay in charge and realize that no one can run this race for you but you.

Taking responsibility does not mean blaming yourself, hating yourself, or beating yourself when you hit hard times and disappointments. It is not your fault when a cycle doesn't work out and you are not pregnant yet.

Taking responsibility means educating yourself, speaking up for yourself, advocating for yourself, believing in yourself. You need to understand and fully realize that you--and only you--are responsible and in charge of your infertility treatments and journey.

582. Prepare to Work Hard: Once you accept the responsibility, it is important to understand that a lot of work may be required to beat infertility.

Infertility treatments require going to lots of appointments, and doing whatever you can to improve your health. This journey takes effort and push. Accepting the hard work involved will make it easier, and hopefully empower you to do what is available to heal your infertility.

583. Prepare To Talk Positively To Yourself Each Day: Starting now, you need to tell yourself every single day that your body can and will get pregnant and give birth.

Say right out loud that your body is healing from infertility, that it is only a temporary condition, and that you are capable, able and strong enough to have a baby.

Repeat over and over again that your body is ready, willing and able to receive and nurture a new life.

It is key that right from the start of this journey, you understand the importance of your self-talk. At this time, you must be your own best friend, your personal cheerleader, your own fertility coach, as you consciously choose to speak words of hope, health and healing to your body.

What you speak aloud and what you speak internally must be positive. No dire pronouncements. No words like, "I'll never get pregnant" or "this won't work out."

You must commit right now that you will speak to your body in a way that
encourages healing, confidence, success, and growth.

All the self-hating, blaming words must end now.

Stop the negative self-talk that the body listens to, and ultimately obeys, on an unconscious level.

Start talking to yourself and your body, both silently and aloud, about the success and healing you are soon going to experience. You need to tell your body that yes, you are going to have a baby. Yes, you are going to be a parent.

Your self-talk needs to be affirm a good and beautiful outcome for your efforts.

Let your body know you love it and you have faith it will find a way to conceive, carry and give birth to a beautiful baby.

Let your ovaries, vagina, kidneys, adrenal glands and liver know that you love them and you believe in their power. Hug yourself, soothe yourself. Stop the voices in your head that call you weak, powerless, sickly, infertile.

Never ever say "this won't work."

When you are feeling down and you can sense that your internal whisperings are going to be negative, stop and envision how lovingly you would talk to a friend in this situation.

Just as you need to talk kindly to yourself, be aware of the words you use when speaking to others about your infertility. Even if you feel discouraged, NEVER EVER say out loud, "I doubt I will get pregnant" or "I don't think this will happen for me."

Repeat: even during difficult times, never let negative words that predict an unhappy outcome for your efforts escape from your lips.

583. Prepare To Never, Never, Never Give Up: Get ready to persevere, persist, and try try again. You need to decide right now that you will jump over every hurdle, cross every river, take every risk, to reach your goal of becoming a parent.

From the start, you need to decide that giving up is not an option-- unless you come to a point that you've found peace with not having biological children and have found another alternative that feels like the right path to take. Persevering means that you will stay with this until you reach your desired outcome.

A note here: If you decide to change your goal, from perhaps giving birth to a biological child to adopting a child, that is not giving up, but making a different, but wonderful, life choice.

Or if you decide having children is not a priority, that is fine too. Persevering is worth it if you desire the goal and quitting feels like the worst option.

584. Prepare To Get Up Fast When You Are Knocked Down By the Word No: You are going to hear the word no sometimes. That is a reality infertility patients need to understand from the very beginning of this journey. Get ready for them and accept it.

If you know the punch is coming, it will still hurt, but maybe not as much as it would if it came unexpectedly and surprised you.

If at times you hear the word, 'no' such as 'no, you are not pregnant' consider the no's nothing more than a missed shot that is a part of this game—a ball that didn't make the hoop this time around and prepare to shoot again.

Prepare to hear many no's on the way to yes. You prepare, not because you are pessimistic or dismal, but so if a 'no' does come your way, it will not knock you down and break your heart so badly that you refuse to try again.

A 'no' should not surprise you, or trip you up, to the point that getting back up to try again feels impossible.

Disappointment and failure is an inherent part of this process. If you expect that disappointment is part of this game, you won't be shocked when something doesn't work out or the nurse calls with a no.

You just have to realize that the disappointments don't mean you are not going to someday arrive at your destination.

It does mean, however, that you will need stamina and perseverance to stay in the infertility game.

But remember: one win in this game means a lifetime World Series status. In this tournament, you don't need ten wins to be a big winner-- you need only one.

You absolutely can't let a temporary loss that comes in the form of a "no" make you so sad that you stop trying.

There will be disappointments during your infertility journey that can make you so sad that they will threaten your ability to get up and try again. The grief and disappointment that can occur during infertility treatments is a threat to a women's ability to plow through the hard times. A person can feel so defeated by a cycle gone wrong that they choose to stop the game altogether and give up the fight. Prepare internally for those hard times, so if and when they do come, you are not knocked out of the game and can re-enter strong and ready to do whatever it takes to improve your chances of giving birth.

While you have every right to want to lock yourself in the house because your neighbor is suddenly pregnant with her fifth child and she chose you to complain to, you do not have the luxury of licking your wounds for too long. You need to be ready to get over it quickly and move on to the next cycle, the next medication, the next clinic, the next acupuncture appointment, the next whatever that is going to move you closer to giving birth to your baby.

You may be one of the lucky ones, and with a bit of medical intervention, wham, you're pregnant. It happens to some women this way. You could very well be one of them. I wish this for you--you certainly deserve it. But if not, it doesn't mean you are not going to get pregnant and have the babies of your dreams. It simply means that you must prepare not to get defeated by the nos.

When you try everything one month, and the nurse calls to say, "no, I'm-sorry- you are not pregnant" you have every right to despair, but then if you want to win and see your dream come true, you must muster your strength, schedule your appointments for the next cycle and try again.

When some cynical doctor tells you he or she doesn't think you can ever get pregnant, you ignore him or her, and get a new doctor who is willing to try a new medication or a new procedure and you try again. You don't get stuck on the negative words of anyone, even authority figures you may have great respect for.

You might hear lots of discouraging talk, read lots of bad statistics, hear lots of no's. You may have despairing moments--it is all part of this process. It is the person who perseveres through these rough times--who keeps making good choices and keeps trying new avenues--who has the best chance of reaching their goal despite the hurdles in the way.

I have a dear friend who underwent four IVFS before she got pregnant and gave birth to her beautiful son. One look at this boy, and you know he was worth it. Just keep in mind, however, what she went through: four IVFS, a few miscarriages, one ovary that wasn't working, and lots of people who said things like, "you did three IVFS. They didn't work. You only have one working ovary. Don't you think it is time to give up."

To continue, you have to accept as part of the process the defeats. The no's cannot be allowed to hold you hostage or push you permanently down into a hole of despair—even when it is your right to feel despair.

Remember: one no, 10 no's, 20 no's, do not have to mean defeat. It only takes one yes in this game, amidst all the nos, to get you what you most want.

You, my strong mother warrior, are a fighter in the ring--you can take some brutal punches and even flat-out knock downs, and still come out a winner.

Remember: your chances of winning increase when you refuse to stay down no matter how devastating the punch.
The more you try, the higher the odds are in your favor. Wallowing too long can leave you stuck, and you could miss key chances to get pregnant. So cry. Scream. Wail. Just don't stay down long. Get up. Try again. Move on.

Prepare for the no's so when they happen, you'll be ready.

585. Prepare to Put Certain Parts of Your Life on Hold: Infertility requires a certain amount of sacrifice. Certain aspects of your life will have to put on hold. Getting pregnant and healing from infertility requires that you make this a priority in your life. It may mean that some of your goals will have to be put on hold, routines will have to be changed, so that all your resources and focus can be on having a baby. You may have to use extra money for treatments that you normally would have used for other things. You might have to put certain house renovations on hold.

You might not be able to commit to as many social functions. You might have to scale back on your work, or use all your vacation time or sick time on infertility treatments. You may need to set aside time at night to prepare healthy foods, instead of watching TV. You might have to be at the clinic early in the morning for blood work, maybe a lot earlier than you used to being out. Sometimes, you may have to change your entire work schedule.

Getting your body ready for conception may mean giving up things and putting in place other things. It may mean a change in lifestyle, a change in eating habits, a change in routine, a change in how you spend your money, a change in where you spend your time, where you vacation, and how you live your life on many levels. These sacrifices will eventually not seem so bad, but preparing for them right from the start will be helpful, so you are not surprised or thrown off course when they happen.

Sacrifice requires keeping your eye on the outcome rather than on the deprivation of the moment.

Sacrifice requires being flexible, and understanding that eventually, you can get back to your normal life and routines, but not right now--right now, your goal of getting pregnant has to take precedence.

Healing from your infertility needs to be a high priority in your life. You can't do infertility treatments and expect to do 1,000 other things at the same time.

When I realized I was in need of some serious healing, any extra money I had went to alternative holistic treatments that complimented my regular healing. I committed to acupuncture weekly. It costs me $40 a treatment. To many of you, that may not seem like a lot of money, but it was enough to mean I couldn't enjoy some small pleasures I once enjoyed, especially when I went a few times a week.

I don't know what sacrifices you will have to make, what money you'll have to spend, what time you will need to put aside.

For me, infertility treatments meant no new clothes, no wild romps of eating anything I wanted. All extra money went to alternative holistic health treatments. Things like new items for the house became distant memories from the past.

We even had a friend live in our basement who paid $400 a month in rent--most of that extra money went towards alternative health treatments to aid in my body's healing.

Expect that, for awhile, certain parts of your life will be put on hold, so that you can give 100 percent of your energy, time and resources to getting pregnant.

586. Prepare to Say Goodbye to Guilt, Shame and Self-Blame: Infertility is not a weakness, a curse, or a sin. Infertility is not something you should feel guilty about. It is not your fault and it certainly doesn't mean you are not meant to be a mother.

Infertility is a temporary physical condition that can be treated and healed. Millions of women once diagnosed with infertility went on to heal and give birth to their babies.

Should a person with a bad cold feel guilty because their nose is running? Doesn't a person with a cold take Vitamin C and rest, knowing that with some orange juice and chicken soup, their nose will eventually stop running and they will return to living without a cold?

Is a person with cancer somehow to blame for the cancer? No, the body sometimes gets on the wrong track, and whether it is a runny nose, an arthritic knee, cancer or acne, we should never blame ourselves for the times when the body goes awry. We are not physically perfect, nor should we expect ourselves to be.

What we are, and what we can expect from ourselves, is the capacity to heal and renew from temporary physical conditions.

Instead of guilt and shame, we need to forgive our body, love our body, be kind and good to our body, and work slowly and lovingly towards healing our body. Illness is in no way a reason to engage in self-hatred. The body cannot be beaten and shamed back into health. It can, however, be loved and soothed back to a healthy state.

Wipe away right now any archaic ideas that you are evil, flawed, or cursed because you are having trouble getting pregnant. You are not a bad person because you have a physical problem with conception.

You are in simply a temporary state of infertility that can be healed. Infertility is a malfunction of the body, just like any illness, and it is no reason to beat yourself up.

Does infertility make you less of a woman? No, no and no. No self-hate allowed. No needless shame or guilt is warranted. You need now to love yourself as much as possible.

What is there to be ashamed of? What is there to feel guilty about? Infertility is not a statement about your character, your worth, your power as a woman, your ability to mother, your maternal calling, your right to be a mother, your childhood, your family history, your ability to mother, or anything else. Infertility is the result of the body straying down an unhealthy track—a track, however, that you can lovingly lead your body away from so that you can ultimately get back on a healthy, vibrant, blooming and yes, fertile track.

Say a goodbye to emotions like guilt and self-hatred because there is no validity to them.

587. Prepare to Hear Some Negative Comments About Infertility Even from the People You Love: Realize and accept right from the start that sometimes you will hear negative comments about your infertility, even from close friends and family.

Not everyone you love will support or understand what you are going through. Some of your dearest and closest friends and relatives may not understand or approve of your pursuing infertility treatments. Others may think it odd that you are having trouble getting pregnant, attributing the problem to something that is "all in your mind." Some may wonder why you want children so badly, labeling you as 'obsessive' or even 'imbalanced.'

Some people may feel it is morally wrong to get medical help to have a baby. Some may not be able to understand at all why you are having trouble getting pregnant. They may blame you and say you are too uptight, anxious or nervous.

Other people might feel uncomfortable seeing someone ardently pursuing something that isn't coming naturally. These are the type of people who may desperately want pancakes for breakfast, but if life serves them up scrambled eggs, they will say thank you, eat them, and never dare to ask for pancakes again. Some people take what they are given, and don't rock the boat by going after what doesn't come naturally or easily.

By pursuing infertility treatments, you are rocking the boat and saying that you are not willing to accept what life has served you.

You want a baby, and if it doesn't come naturally, well, then you will do whatever modern medicine has at its disposal to make this baby come alive.

That freaks some people out--and you need to prepare and know that, so you can get ready for some criticism and disapproval. You need to carefully select whom you will tell about your infertility treatments, and who you share information with.

There are some people who already have children, and maybe all they dream about is a quiet weekend away without the hard work of caring for kids. So to them, they really don't get what your intense longing is all about. They've sadly lost sight of the immense beauty and gift children are, and because they have lost sight, they can't imagine what the big deal is and why you seem so determined to have a baby. They may even try to convince you to let this go and stay childless. Beware of these cynics, who may simply be just exhausted parents in disguise or parents who have lost the ability to see the joy in raising kids.

Others may not see you as "the mother type" because they can't imagine you in a role they haven't seen you in yet. Ignore them. They obviously don't know who you really are and what you are capable of.

If they can't see your maternal abilities, that is their lack of understanding. These are the same people who will someday go on and on about what a great mother you are.

There are a host of other discouraging, negative comments people may send your way. To some older friends and relatives, the whole "science-making-a-baby-thing" can seem weird, odd, freakish and scary.

Don't let all these negative comments in.

Screen carefully who you let be part of this process. Only let in friends and family who are positive, and who can ultimately see a good result for you. People who say things like, "Maybe God doesn't want you to have a baby" need to be shut out during this time. Since when did they get the right to speak for God? Don't talk to negative people about your dream of having a child.

Try not to be angry at these type of comments--forgive those you love, but don't let your infertility become a topic of conversation with them.

If you are prepared for the negative comments, they will not throw you off course so easily or make you limp at the 'surprise attacks.' Instead, you will be cautious and aware of who you talk to about infertility. You'll also understand that nothing they say or feel about this matters.

You'll realize that whatever negative shots are thrown your way come from ignorance, fear, misunderstanding or just plain stupidity. Don't let it get to you. Don't let the comments penetrate. Shake them off and keep walking towards your heart's true desire.

588. Prepare To Get Organized: Getting organized is an important part of this journey. Purchase a date book or a blackberry where you can keep track of all your appointments.

Keep a notebook, preferably with pockets, where you can jot down any and all information that might help you with your treatments.
Helpful ideas, information from holistic practitioners, doctors and nurses, can all be stored in this notebook.

The more organized you are, the smoother this whole process will go.

What helped me was a daily calendar at-a-glance appointment book where I kept all phone numbers and appointments related to my infertility treatments.

I also had a big green notebook where I kept all information I gathered from books, magazine articles, television specials, on topics related to infertility, such as infertility medications, foods to help heal infertility. Anything I read or heard that might be of help to me all went into that notebook.
Having all my information in one place helped me follow-up on things I learned. Infertility treatments can be a bit like starting a new job: a lot is expected and there is little time to adjust. You may need to organize what you will eat each day--no more 'I-have-nothing-in-the-house-so-sugar/fast food/low quality food/ will have to due.'

Any vitamins or herbs you will be taking need also to be organized. If you are doing several cleanses in preparation of fertility treatments, you'll need to organize these also.

In addition to keeping track and being on time for all your appointments with the infertility clinic, you'll also need to keep track of any appointments with alternative practitioners, such as chiropractors or acupuncturists.

If you are also planning to add some stress-relieving type of exercises into your daily routine, you'll also need to do some time management and scheduling to make this happen.

You'll also need to organize foods, snacks and containers for these items, so that you always have on hand healthy foods, instead of being forced to eat junk food or fast foods, because you are starving and nothing is available. That might also mean preparing foods at night for the next day, washing fruits or vegetables and putting them in bags, or cooking several healthy meals ahead of time and freezing them.

When I began to seriously understand the role I needed to play in my own healing, I had to schedule time for light swimming, time to prepare healthy foods the night before work and acupuncture appointments.

Being well-organized will also help you when you feel emotionally shaky and unsure of your next step. Knowing what you need to do tomorrow can help keep you on track moving forward towards your goal.

589. Prepare to Switch Gears--and Switch Gears Often: Successfully coping with infertility can sometimes mean knowing when it is time to switch gears and try something new.

Switching gears can mean knowing when it is time to change doctors, try a different medication, or incorporate some holistic healing into your treatments.

Infertility treatments require the ability to shift gears and change tracks when the one you are on isn't working. It requires bending, twisting and contorting as the path unfolds. Being prepared to switch gears means being flexible and welcoming change when need is needed. It means trying new ways of healing when they are presented to you. It means not clinging to a certain doctor or a certain medication that isn't working.

This journey is not always Step A to Step B, it is sometimes Step A to Step N to Step Z back to Step C. Get your dancing shoes on and be ready for the trapeze act that will sometimes be required of you.

Don't stay stuck thinking there is only one way to reach your goal--if that path is not working, switch gears and be ready to go down a new path if you need to.

590. Prepare To Tap Into Your Power: To endure some of the challenges of infertility, you need to tap into your power.

While you cannot control or determine the outcome of your fertility journey, you do have some measure of power. You have the power to make choices, power to persevere, power to pray to God, power to believe against all odds, power to think positively, power to phone a friend who is positive and encouraging, power to read a book or listen to music that inspires, power to exercise, power to communicate, power to connect to nature, power to eat healthy foods, power to get up the next day, power to walk forward, power to sing, power to dance--power to envision ourselves in a life with the children we most desire.

Get ready to tap into all the power that is yours, that God has given all humans, and that can help you as you strive towards this goal. You have power over what you eat, what you drink, and what you say out loud and to yourself.

You have the power to endure pain when you have to. You may have to endure shots twice a day for several weeks, and you may have to do this even if you think right now you could never endure shots. I am the biggest chicken on the planet--a person who can tolerate very little pain--and after awhile, the shots seemed like no big deal to me. If I can do it, you can too. Trust me on this one. You are have more power than you realize. You will be amazed at the power within you as you walk through infertility. Get ready to embrace it.

591. Prepare For The Hard times By Creating Happiness Zones in Your Life: You need from the very start of your infertility journey to create happiness zones that will give you some comfort and joy when the going gets tough.

A happiness zone is anything that nudges you gently over to a road of happiness, and shields you, even for a few minutes, from feelings of sadness, anxiety, anger and nervousness. A happiness zone can be a place you love to visit, time spent with a person who always leaves you feeling happy, a favorite picture, a game, hobby or a pet.

The more happiness zones you create in your life, the easier the hard times will be to endure. A happiness zone can be a weekly date with a friend, a singing or acting class, a knitting group, a book club, buying yourself flowers every Tuesday, taking yourself to a weekly picnic, or buying a fish tank, a cat or a plant.

Set up routines so you have pleasant experiences to look forward to each week. Is there a beautiful park nearby that you can take a walk at once a week? A place in your yard you can sit 15 minutes a day and enjoy the sunshine?

Have videos, music and books readily available that make you laugh and feel positive. Surround yourself with music that transport you back to happy times in your life.

Ask yourself: what makes me happy? Include these in your life more often! What can you do to make breakfast more enjoyable? Your drive to work? Your lunch hour or break time? Evenings at home? Saturday mornings?

Break it down by the hour if you have to—what would elevate your feelings of joy? It can be anything, from taking out your collection of childhood teddy bears and displaying them in the living room, to doing karaoke once a week with a new group of friends, to reading a chapter of the Bible daily.

Think about what made you happy when you were a child, a teenager and a young adult. Get ready to tap into the most ancient parts of yourself and start including those long-forgotten activities in your life.

In whatever ways you can, add fun and comfort to your home, your routines, and your life. These will lift you up as you walk this road.

592. Prepare to Research the Subject of Infertility: Take the time to research and learn about the reasons why you may be having trouble getting pregnant. Visit the library and bookstore. Phone holistic and alternative practitioners and have a chat. Ask questions. Read blogs on infertility. Exchange ideas with others who have successfully beaten infertility. Investigate what new medications and research is out there. You never know what nugget of information will turn be the one to turn the key to your body's healing.

593. Prepare to Banish the 'No-You-Don't-Deserve-That Monster' Who May Lurk In Your Subconscious: Inside many of us, there lives a little no monster who is always telling us 'no'. The little no-monster wants to punish and deny us.

The little no-monster will say, 'no, you can't have that!' 'no you can't do that!' 'no you don't deserve that!' 'no someone like you will never get that!'

If you are going to harness all your power to make a baby, you need to set the 'no-monster' straight right from the beginning, and let it know 'yes, I can have a baby' 'yes, I deserve a baby' 'yes, I am capable of giving birth.'

Tell the no-monster 'yes I can get pregnant', 'yes my body is strong enough to conceive a child and hold it safely for nine months', 'yes someone like me will have a baby' 'yes, I deserve this to work out.'

The no-monster will remind you of all the times in your life you tried and failed. It will remind you of all the times you really, really wanted something and you failed to get it. It will remind you of all the things you didn't achieve and all the people who hurt you. It will say over and over again that you are not the kind of person who ever gets what you want. It will tell you that you are a failure.

It will tell you that woman with your type ofpersonality/childhood/family history/experiences/ can't do this.

You need to tell the no-monster to SHUT UP AND GO AWAY!

You need to squash that voice, argue it away, and put your inner yes master to work.

Because inside you also lives a 'yes master.' The 'yes master' believes in you and knows you can win. This 'yes master' knows very well that you are very capable of having a baby.

Allow this 'yes master' to scream right out loud that yes, you deserve a baby. Yes, you will get what you want. Yes, you can achieve what you set out to achieve. The yes-master will remind you of all those times in your life when you worked hard and achieved your goal.

It will remind you that miracles happen everyday, and people who never imagined they could get pregnant somehow end up having beautiful babies.

It will remind you that although your road may be long and hard, you can still reach your destination. The 'yes master' will encourage you to never give up. It will help you tap into the strong, courageous part of you who is able to step up to the plate and do whatever it takes to win.

Let the 'yes-master' be your friend through this ordeal, and tell the 'no-monster' to shove off.

594. Prepare to receive: Becoming pregnant is, in part, an act of receiving. Being open to conceiving a baby is the act of receiving a precious gift—a gift you very much deserve.

So starting now, get yourself in the habit of receiving. Make receiving something you feel very comfortable with. Buy yourself small gifts every week, so that receiving becomes something you get used to.

Write down all the good things you've received in your life, things you willingly allowed yourself to receive, things that came to you just because you are a human and good things can sometimes flow to us if we allow ourselves to receive it. Think of all the things you easily and freely receive in your life, such as air, gravity, sunshine, and a womb where your child can grow.

Wrap small presents and give them to yourself as a reminder that you, as a human being on this earth, have a right to receive good things.

Remember: you don't need to be perfect to receive good things.

You can be flawed, imperfect, and still be worthy of receiving good things.

Sometimes you will receive good things just because.

Sometimes you will receive good things because you worked hard for them.

Sit outside and allow yourself to receive the warmth of the sun. Sit under a tree and let yourself receive its cooling shade. Sit by the ocean and let yourself receive the calming sound of the waves.

Each week, take note of all the wonderful things you received that week--from a text that brightened your day, to a hug or kiss, to a good night's sleep, to a glimpse of something unexpected that just made you happy.

Let the emotion and experience of receiving begin to feel natural to you.

595. Prepare to Change the Way You Care for your Body: Healing from infertility requires taking care of your body in a new way that you may have never done before. You may need to entirely change the way you eat, cook and experience food in your life. You may have to change your sleep schedule, exercise routines, and how you use food to cope with emotions and during times of fun and celebration.

You may have to pay closer attention to what you put on your skin, and around your body and in your environment, which can then enter your body. You may have to spend a lot more time preparing foods then you did in the past.

The upside is, not only will you be taking steps to heal your infertility, but you most likely will also start feeling healthier in every other way too.

596. Prepare As If You Were A Professional Runner Training For A Race: While going through infertility, consider yourself a runner training for a race. Professional runners are aware that there are many obstacles that can come up during a race and they prepare ahead of time for them.

Successful runners develop the trait of resilience, which gives them the power to bounce back from setbacks. They acknowledge the setback, but quickly move past it so they can focus on the goal ahead.

They know the importance of developing mental toughness and strength so they can continue running, regardless of the conditions, distractions, and emotions they experience during a race.

A successful runner develops the ability to keep moving forward towards their goal, even when there are no immediate signs of winning or even being closer to the finish line. They develop an inner voice that says, 'I can do this. I have the resources inside of me to succeed.' They keep running towards their goal, even when the finish line seems impossible to reach. Some runners write positive sayings on their arms or water bottles so they have a motivational thought to carry them through. Some runners keep themselves going by visualizing how it will feel to get to the finish line and win the race.

While going through your infertility treatments, you plan ahead and prepare a strategy to follow even during the rough times. You develop a mental toughness, so you can bounce back from disappointment, whether or not anyone is cheering you on or believes you can win.

You follow your plan of action, even when your goal seems elusive or faraway. You keep listening to that positive inner voice that says: 'yes, you can get pregnant' even when the finish line is nowhere in sight.

597. Prepare To Be Self-Disciplined: Infertility treatments require a lot of self-discipline. It takes self-discipline not to delve into a box of donuts when you are stressed. It takes self-discipline to get to the clinic for blood work and ultrasound at 6 a.m. It takes self-discipline to go to bed early. It takes self-discipline to keep going to a myofascial release expert or a chiropractor week after week.

It takes self-discipline to remember to buy some walnuts and pumpkin seeds, put them in snack bags and bring them to work to eat during break, instead of grabbing something fast from the vending machine. It takes self-discipline to walk each morning to relieve stress.

Self-discipline means following through on what you start. Self-discipline means getting to your appointments on time. Self-discipline means continuing with treatments and foods that can heal you—even when they are inconvenient and boring. Being self-disciplined will help you stay consistent. It will help you say no when you want to say yes. Or say yes when you wish you could say no.

598. Prepare To Connect To Your Body: Stop hating your curves, dreading your 'time of the month' and disliking the shape and size of your breasts. No, they are NOT too big/too small/ too whatever. They are just perfect.

Stop hating the smells that come from your vagina or underarms.

Stop. Just stop.

Its time to start embracing your womanly, feminine body.

This includes your menstrual cycle, your pubic hair, your shapely (or not so shapely) backside.

Start honoring your period. No bad mouthing it, please. It is part of the birth cycle. Stop denying it and suppressing it. Love it and appreciate it.

Your body, in all its amazing womanliness, is trying to do its best for you. Say thank you to it. Give it a big hug. Show some gratitude.

How To Cope With The Emotions That Come From Suffering With Infertility:

599. Anger: Infertility is hell (I said it before and I will say it again) and if you feel angry about the whole thing, you have every right to feel that way.

We feel angry when we are frustrated and unable to get what we want.

Anger is an emotion that is often a combination of feeling powerless, afraid and hurt.

Anger sometimes appears in the form of resentment, irritability, rage, animosity, and bitterness.

In Chinese medicine it is believed that anger affects the liver, which is a key organ in infertility. The more you release the toxins in your liver, the less your body will be able to hold onto anger.

There are also alternative/holistic therapies that can help release anger, such as craniosacral/myofascial therapy, acupuncture, and homeopathy. Massage and trauma release can also help release anger. Swimming can be a safe way to release anger. I started swimming when I began infertility treatments, and once found myself sobbing after a very intense swim. I didn't know why I was crying, but I sensed my body was releasing pent-up anger.

Spending time in nature, sitting by the ocean, are also ways to release anger.

When you begin to feel anger, try to do one thing that gives you a feeling of control in your life, such as juicing a green drink, saying a positive affirmation, or going to an acupuncture appointment.

Close your eyes and picture the part of you that is angry and ask that part of you: what can I give you right now that will help you feel better?

Let your inner child know you will help her have the baby she so desires. Comfort her. Ask her: what is it you want honey? Then listen closely for the answers.

Remember: anger is a secondary emotion. There is something you feel before you feel angry. Try to identify what emotions you feel before you reach anger.

When you begin to feel angry, say: 'I am powerful. I am powerful and able to get what I want.'

Do something creative that gives your anger a chance leave your body and take another form outside of yourself.

Anger does not have to trap you into a helpless state that leaves your body stressed. Acknowledge it, give yourself something that it needs, and release it when you can.

600. Jealousy: Jealousy is an emotion everyone feels at one time or another, regardless of our circumstances and situations in life. We all feel jealous when we see someone with something we desperately want, but don't have. It is easy to feel jealous of women who have children. Don't feel guilty about experiencing this emotion. Jealousy often comes from a perceived scarcity in an area of your life. So rather than seeing other people's babies as a slap in the face, begin to see it as a cue that 'if it is possible for them, it is possible for me.'

The next time you see a mother with her children and you feel jealous, say to yourself: if it could happen to her, it could happen to me.

Think of it this way: her success today mirrors the potential for your success tomorrow.

When you hear of a baby shower or find out a friend is pregnant, it means that pregnancy and birth are conditions possible in our world—possible for them and possible for you.

Realize that just because you don't have something today doesn't mean you won't have it tomorrow.

Try, (I know how hard this is) to keep a vision of a tomorrow where you have the babies you deserve.

Repeat: 'There is enough to go around.' 'There is enough for everybody.' 'I too can have what I want.' 'I will have a baby too.'

When you see a baby, repeat the words: 'babies are born, babies are here, babies are everywhere, and my baby is coming too.' Or: 'this just proves that babies are always coming and my baby is coming too.'

Feeling robbed and jealous are not emotions that just disappear overnight. Nor should you feel guilty when you experience them. Just keep reminding yourself that every baby you see is a reminder that babies are born everyday—and one of these days it could very well be your baby that is born! Keep a note on your refrigerator that says: "There is enough for everybody! There is enough for me! Lots of women have babies and I will have one too!"

601. Frustration: Frustration is a common emotion for those coping with infertility. It is frustrating to want something very badly and not be able to get it.

Frustration is an emotion linked to feeling helpless and powerless, a combination of feeling disappointed and angry. So taking some type of action, such as doing something new to heal your body, can be a remedy for this emotion. When you take action, you are reminding yourself that you are not powerless.

Remind yourself each day that you are not helpless, you are not powerless, and that your body is capable and able to heal if given the right tools.

For me, prayer gave me a feeling of power and trust in God that I needed when my own efforts felt blocked or thwarted.

When I was frustrated, I would write a list of what I was going to do the next day to help my body heal from infertility. Making that list gave me a sense of power because—I was doing something to help myself heal from infertility.

I was showing myself that I could find solutions to my problems and that with the right steps, things could work out for me.

Taking action and responsibility is what will help alleviate feelings of frustration.

602. Fear: Fear is an emotion that sometimes accompanies infertility. You may fear never getting pregnant or you may fear some of the procedures and tests you have to go through.

According to Chinese medicine, excessive or prolonged fear drains the kidneys and suppresses Qi energy in the body. Fear is an emotion that can wreak havoc with your hormones.

Fear is an emotion that is caused by the belief that something is dangerous, likely to cause us pain or is a threat. To cope with fear, name it, face it and acknowledge it. Go within and write down your fears concerning infertility: do you fear not getting what you want? Or getting what you want? Once you name your fear, you then can begin to find ways to calm your nervous system and let it know you are safe.

Remember: never let the fear of striking out keep you from playing the game.

603. Sadness or Grief: Feeling grief-stricken and extremely sad are normal emotions that infertility patients often experience. Never feel ashamed or weak because of your sadness. You have a right to it. Sometimes, you just have to give yourself permission to feel sad, while at the same time, do whatever you can to keep the endorphins or "happy chemicals" in your body moving.

How To Cope With The Ups and Downs of Infertility Treatments

604. How do you not go crazy when you run into an old friend who has three beautiful kids and just announced she is happily pregnant with her fourth?

How do you keep going, when the shots, the appointments, the painful tests, seem never ending?

How do you persevere when the nurse calls again with another, 'no, I'm sorry' message.

Sometimes, not being able to get pregnant is nothing short of torture, anguish, a raw clawing frustration, because what is natural is not coming naturally.

There were times during my infertility treatments when I was hysterical, depressed, unable to be consoled.

This is no easy time and no easy task.

There will be times when you will rightly feel very angry, frustrated and even downright hopeless. My guess is that you are a lot stronger than you think you are, but feelings are feelings and sometimes they are just there and can't be ignored.

Here's what five years of infertility treatments taught me about coping with the ups and downs that accompany this difficult and trying process.

605. Accept the Fact That Infertility Is Sometimes Going To Be Heartbreaking: Yes, enduring infertility is hard. Very very hard. Wicked hard (if I dare flashback to my 1980s youth.)

Once you accept that is hard, you can go from there. This is not an easy road, but you are inherently strong enough and capable enough to handle the difficulty.

Once you accept the difficulty of this process, you won't be surprised at the work and perseverance sometimes needed to get through this.

Accepting that it will be hard means you will accept the work, and have the patience and perseverance to get through it. And, most importantly, you won't be shocked when you hit some very hard bumps in the road.

606. Accept That Some Days You Are Just Going To Fall Apart: There are going to be days when it all gets too much. The unfairness of what you are going through, the longing for a child that continues to be unfulfilled, the raw pain of seeing a world filled with pregnant women and babies, and you somehow denied that joy, will all get too much. When that happens, you might collapse into bed, cry uncontrollably, rage at your husband, flip out at the next friend who tells you to just relax.

You won't always behave appropriately, you might do unproductive things. Sometimes you might just feel like the pain of it all is going to kill you.

Knowing ahead of time that this might happen won't relieve you of the pain, but it might help you remember that thousands of women who experienced infertility also have had bad days like this—and thousands of them now have children. Eventually, many of them got pregnant and gave birth, despite heartbreaking disappointments.
That lady you walked by in the supermarket with the adorable kids who made your heart ache? She very well could have been an infertility patient once upon a time.

Know this: you may be crying hysterically today because you are not pregnant, and a year or two from now, you might be spending your day taking care of your sweet baby.

607. In Your Darkest Moments, Remember What Choices Are Still Available to You: During the moments when you feel you can't take anymore, ask yourself this question: what is one thing I can do today that will move me one step closer to my goal? You got a call and the news was bad: no, you are not pregnant. In that moment of complete disappointment, stop and ask yourself: what is one positive action I can do right now to help me get one step closer to having a baby? Before you fall apart, before you start crying, ask yourself this one question and immediately take a step towards this positive action.

608. Never Forget the Link Between the Choices You Make and the Consequences That Follow: It is easy to feel helpless during infertility treatments. It is easy to feel like you have no control over the outcome, and to some degree, that is true. However, you do have choices that are under your control.

Everyday, you can make choices that can either empower your body or debilitate your body. While you cannot guarantee the outcome of your infertility journey, you can improve your chances by making good choices. You can choose to consume less sugar and caffeine, and as a result, your health could slightly improve.

Choose to walk 15 minutes a day, and you may lose weight, which in turns helps balance your hormones.

609. Take Control Of What You Can Control: To cope with all the things that happen during infertility that are out of your control, learn to take control of what you can control. You have control over what enters your mouth and what you put on our skin. You have control over what type of water you drink, what types of cleaning chemicals you use in your home and yard, and what types of holistic healing you bring into your life. During your moments of despair, grab hold of what is still under your control and do the best, most positive, healing action available to you. What you can control, control well.

610. Just Say No To Denial: To beat infertility, you have to face head on the problems you are experiencing. During treatments, don't allow yourself to go into denial if that will inhibit your ability to make choices that will help heal your body. Do you have the right doctor—one who is proactive, open to suggestions and ready to try different medications? Or are you ignoring that nagging feeling that your doctor is not on the right track with your treatments? Have you been on the same medication for a long time and it is not working? Come on, be truthful, look straight at it, no more hiding the truth from yourself. Is there a condition your body is suffering from that you are not paying attention to, such as exhausted adrenal glands, a parasitic infestation, a lack of sunlight or sleep, or chemicals in your system that need to be released? Face it, name it, look straight at it, and then work to fix it. Denial is not your friend in beating infertility.

611. Make it Easy To Hope By Physically Showing Your Complete Belief That You Will Someday Have a Baby: It is important that you physically showcase and manifest in some way your complete and utter belief that you will have a baby. Put some physical manifestations of hope around you, i.e. a stuffed animal you will give your child, a photo album that says baby's first year, a toy.

By doing this, you will be moving past your present reality into a new reality--a reality where you absolutely know and believe that your baby is on the way to you.

I hung a poster in my kitchen entitled "Relax...God is in Charge." Reading this poster always gave me a sweet, calming sense of peace. If there are sayings that give you feelings of hope, joy and peace, put them in places where you can read them daily and let your body experience the positive force of these words. Put symbols, pictures, quotes in your everyday life that make it easy for your mind to float over to the realm of hope.

612. Listen To Your Body: Ssh, listen. What is your body trying to tell you? During infertility treatments, it is important that you start listening for the subtle and sometimes not-so-subtle messages your body is trying to send you.

Listen to that inner voice that knows what your body needs to heal. Don't shut this voice up--it may be of great help to you.

If suddenly you get the urge that your body needs a certain food or treatment, honor that inclination. You know more than you consciously realize about what your body needs to get pregnant.
Keep a journal where you ask your body questions like: why are you having trouble getting pregnant? What can I do to help you get pregnant? and let your deep subconscious speak and reveal what it needs.

613. Keep Reminders in Your Home of the Times When Seemingly Impossible Dreams Came True and You Got What You Really Wanted: Hang diplomas and awards from school. Frame letters and cards from family and friends. Call it: My Wall of Happy Ever After or The Wall That Proves Dreams Come True.

Display achievements in your life that resulted from a lot of hard work, along good things that came for no reason at all. Display photos of a wonderful vacation, a picture of the first house or car you ever bought, a gift from a friend, your wedding photos, a love letter, a seashell-- anything that reminds you of times in your life when dreams you worried were not attainable came true. Look at these reminders often. Write the story of how you met your true love, found your lovable dog, or got to experience something you never thought you were going to be able to experience.

614. Memo To You: You Are Not A Victim: While you are being treated for infertility, remind yourself that you are not a victim. A victim has no choices. A victim cannot change their situation. A victim is forever stuck with the same problem. A victim has to rely on someone to save them. A victim is passive. A victim is without hope. You, on the other hand, can do things to change your situation.

You can...

--Ask your doctor questions, change doctors if your doctor is not aggressive enough or fails to listen to you or doesn't try every possible procedure and every possible medication to get you pregnant.

--Try a new medicine or research medicines and ask to be put on a different medicine than one you are on that is not working.

--Request every test available.

--Eliminate white flour products and trans fats from your diet.

--Eat lots of romaine lettuce, spinach, chicory, and other good-for-you green vegetables.

--Go to your primary care doctor or allergist and request tests to determine if you have any food allergies that are weakening your body. Armed with this information, you can stop all foods that are not promoting your body's optimum health.

--Do a parasite cleanse and get unwanted parasites out of your system.

--Do a yeast cleanse and balance the flora in your system.

--Do a liver cleanse and rid your liver of toxins.

--Have your thyroid checked.

--Get several colon cleanses that will release toxins and help improve your elimination

--Start walking, singing, deep breathing, gardening and drawing, to release stress.

--Find an acupuncturist who understands infertility and begin weekly, twice or three times weekly treatments to strengthen your chi, or life energy.

--Keep a journal and express and release negative feelings.

--Pray. Then pray again. Then pray some more.

--Talk to people who are positive, supportive and believe in your ability to have a baby.

--Listen to healing music or music with positive messages.

--Paint the walls in your home beautiful colors that make you happy.

--Stop watching TV programs that are frightening or upsetting and instead start watching shows that make you laugh.

--Avoid situations that drain your energy.

--Visualize the day your baby is born.

-- Speak about your journey to having a baby with confidence, optimism, and total belief.

--Get rid of the doctor who doesn't act fast enough, aggressive enough, or just keeps telling you to relax.

--Find a doctor who answers all your questions, listens to your ideas and suggestions and who is aggressive in their treatment.

--Choose an infertility clinic with a fantastic success record.

--Go to a top notch chiropractor and get your spine aligned, and wear good walking shoes that doesn't throw your spine and hips out of alignment.

-- Find a myofascial release specialist who specializes in trauma release to help you let go of emotional blocks or trauma in your body.

615. Remind Yourself That Your Infertility is Temporary: When you are having a bad week, remind yourself that infertility is not a permanent condition. Remind yourself that infertility is a temporary condition. Temporary, temporary, temporary. Put that word right in your head: temporary. Infertility is temporary. Temporary.

From day one, start looking at infertility as a temporary condition. Infertility is not and should not be considered a permanent condition. Start seeing your body as capable of healing from infertility. Stop viewing this as a permanent condition that your body can't escape from.

If you were suffering with a toothache, would you imagine yourself permanently having this toothache or would you think: 'I have a toothache, I'm going to go to the dentist and be treated for it, and it will be gone'.

See your body in a state of positive change heading towards conception and pregnancy—with infertility as only a temporary stage you are passing through.

Even if you are officially diagnosed with 'unexplained infertility', it is only a temporary label explaining what your body is experiencing at this moment.

It is not a lifetime sentence.

The human body changes minute to minute, based on factors like, what we eat, what forms of healing we allow ourselves to experience, the environment we put ourselves in and elements we use to connect physically and emotionally to our healthiest self.

Our body is always in the midst of change and always capable of change. A woman weighing 200 pounds is labeled "grossly obese' by her doctor, but if she begins exercising and eating nutritious food, a year later, that label is no longer applicable because she made different choices that changed the state of her body.

Consider your body as the composite of many ingredients that result in a recipe, which is the state of your health. If you change the ingredients, you change the recipe.

Your body has the power to heal and change from an ill and infertile state to a fertile healthy state.

616. Keep the 'Happy Chemicals' In Your Brain Flowing: Work hard to make sure the 'happy' chemicals in your brain are working at their maximum capacity. Infertility can be devastating to your emotional self, so try to counteract it by revving up the happy-chemicals your brain. Exercise gently, eat lots of green vegetables, get lots of sleep, reduce your coffee intake and take extra folic acid.

Research has shown that embracing a positive new goal stimulates the release of dopamine, believing in yourself triggers serotonin. Putting yourself around people you trust releases oxytocin. Sniffing vanilla and lavender releases endorphins. Knitting or sewing can give you feelings similar to meditation. To enhance your positive experiences, write them down.

617. Remind Yourself Of What Helped You Cope with Challenging Times in the Past: What kept you emotionally strong and able to cope during hard times in your past? What helped pull you back from despair? When you were sad, where did you seek comfort and find relief?

How did you keep yourself motivated and forward-moving during the rough patches in your life?

Spend some time recalling how you dealt with challenging situations in the past, and be prepared to tap back into these sources of strength.

For me, what helped me to cope was my reliance on God. God has always My faith reminded me that God can help us conquer even the most impossible situations.

I often reminded myself that God could give me strength to do anything, even when in my own human strength, it did not feel possible.
I often thought to myself: if God could open the Red Sea, or shut the mouths of lions, or save three young boys from a fiery furnace, then this is very possible for me. Now ask yourself: what helped me cope in the past that I can tap back into when I need it?

618. When You Are Going Through A Rough Patch in Infertility Treatments, Turn It Into A Happy-Ever-After Story: When you are going through a particularly rough time, write a story about the challenges you are facing, but write into your story a happy ending with you giving birth to a child. Project yourself into a future where you finally get pregnant and have the baby you dream of. When you endure a cycle that is grueling, sit down and write about it—just make sure to add the happiest outcome you can imagine. Don't worry if the story is well-written, grammatically correct, or even makes sense—as long as you write a happy ending to it.

619. Switch It Up: Switch it up: you are not a woman without a baby— you are a woman preparing to be a mother. If anyone asks if you are pregnant, don't say no, instead tell them you are are 'prematernal.'

You are not a infertility patient—you are a mother preparing her body to incubate her baby who is coming soon.

You are not a woman who didn't get pregnant this month—you are a woman whose child is going to be born 10, 11, 12 months from now.

Instead of calling yourself 'infertile' call yourself pre-pregnant.

620. Believe and Act With Complete Confidence In A Positive Future: Write letters to your future child, start planning a Disney vacation for five years in the future. Act as if the arrival of your child is inevitable.

621. Adopt a 'Next, Next, Next' Attitude: I once had a wise friend tell me that in to succeed, you can't let yourself get stuck when you have a goal. When things go wrong, instead of wasting time wallowing think: next, next, next. When things are difficult, take the next action, make the next choice, do the next right thing.

If your doctor tells you there is no hope, get another doctor. Next.

If the medication you have been taking doesn't seem to be working, ask to try another medication. Next.

The nurse called and told you your cycle didn't work out. You reschedule for your next cycle. Next.

If what you are doing doesn't seem to be working, start doing some research and try something new. Next.

Don't get stuck no matter what. Take a next-next-next approach and keep going.

622. Develop a Strategy: When you are fighting something, you need a strategy to beat your opponent and win. That means understanding who your enemy is and what is needed to defeat it.

It means knowing your strengths and weaknesses, what obstacles might come in your way, and how you will overcome these obstacles.

During my infertility, I spent a lot of time researching how the body works, and what can set the body on a wrong track. I began to understand the "enemies" of my fertility, or the places where my body was weak and needed help.

You need a strategy for how you will eat, how you will give your body the amount of sleep, water and sunshine it needs, how you will release your stress and trauma, and how you will maximize the strength and health of every organ in your body.

Having a strategy with a clear path and a series of steps can help keep you on the right track, even during the rough times.

623. Every Night, Ask Yourself: What Is One thing I Can Do Tomorrow to Improve My Chances of Having a Baby?: Make a list each night before bed of what you can do the next day to move you one step closer to getting pregnant. Note what you have to prepare that night so you can accomplish your goals the next day.

When you wake up, look at your list from the night before and get to work. Use this list as a guide for how you are going to stay on track that day. For example, can you have green tea on hand for the drive into work, instead of the big coffee you used to start your day with?

624. Don't Give Any Medical Professional Too Much Power When it Comes To Your Treatment: Always get a second opinion. Remind yourself that doctors are not always right. Just because one doctor is discouraging or sees no hope for you doesn't mean you have to take their diagnosis as a final statement on your fertility. Just because one medical professional sees your situation a certain way doesn't mean it is the only truth or your condition. Get a second, third, or a fourth opinion.

Once, I had a very well-respected doctor, named as the best infertility doctor in New England, tell me that my eggs were "bottom of the barrel" and it was unlikely I would ever get pregnant again, and that I should consider using an egg donor if I wanted a second child.

For a few minutes, her words totally knocked me down and out.

I felt broken, shrunken, put in my place, defeated. I wanted a child with my own eggs, thank you!

Not that it isn't a great option for many, but for me at that time, it wasn't something I was comfortable with or willing to do. On the way home from that hope-shrinking, earth-shattering encounter, I stopped at a natural food market and started looking through books. I guess without knowing it, I was searching for some glimmer of hope. I found a second wind in a book written by Christine Northrup.

In it, she wrote about how in other cultures, women in their 40s become pregnant without a lot of problems, and that some of the infertility problems in our culture could be because of our cultural attitudes toward aging. This information gave me some of hope I needed at that moment.

When I got home, I was still feeling really shaken up, so I phoned my mother. Thank God for my mother, who immediately told me to get rid of that doctor and get another one! My mother was absolutely right. During my meeting with this doctor, she had refused to answer any of my questions from a list I sent her weeks before our meeting, refused to consider trying another medication, (which my next doctor did try and it worked) and seemed more concerned with not being bothered with too many questions, than really helping me get pregnant.

The doctor I chose next was a wonderful man, who listened to me, took the time to answer all 21 of my questions, and agreed with me that it was time to try a more aggressive medication. He even had selected the same medication I had requested my other doctor try with me. I wonder now: why didn't that other doctor want to try me on a new medication? Why did she refuse to even consider it?

Was she afraid that if I didn't get pregnant, her success rate would drop, and her ranking as the best infertility doctor in the area would be threatened? Did she advocate egg donation because she thought it would up my chances of becoming pregnant—and, in turn, make her statistics look better? Was there some financial or professional benefit to her if I went with her suggestion, rather than to continue trying with my own eggs?

Was I simply a pain-in-the-butt patient she wanted to get rid of because I was too intense, showed too much emotion, worked her nurses too hard, and asked too many questions?

Whatever her motive, she almost stopped my son from being born. If I was willing to keep trying, why did she want to persuade me not to try? Was she really thinking of my best interests? Nope. And that is why you can never take one doctor's pronouncement as some type of irrefutable gospel.

Please, don't get sucked in just because some magazine names a doctor as one of the best in the region—they may be doing things to falsely up their statistics or hiring a publicist to market and promote themselves to the media behind the scenes. Or maybe they simply bought an ad in the magazine to garner this rank.

Please don't be deceived because your doctor is loved by everyone you know—if they are giving up on you and you do not want to give up—go find a doctor willing to fight for you and your future child. My doctor was extremely popular, which shows that you have to judge a doctor on what they are doing for you, not for everyone else.

The next doctor I had, who worked in the very same clinic, was completely different--proving that there are doctors who respect their patients and who are willing to go the extra mile.

I wonder now what would have happened if my mother hadn't given me such good advice to get rid of this doctor? What if I had been a more compliant personality and I believed the good doctor, deeming her to be an expert that "knows better"? Well, today I would not have my son.

My gorgeous beautiful son from my own bottom-of-the-barrel eggs.

Someday, I'm going to send this doctor a picture of my beautiful son, and in blazing letters across the picture I am going to write: "THIS IS WHAT BOTTOM OF THE BARREL LOOKS LIKE."

So don't listen. Shut those bad guys up. Dump them. Move on to someone who believes in you.

If a doctor tells you to give up hope, thank them kindly and find a new doctor who is willing to investigate your particular condition and get to the root of the problem. Ultimately, you have to be your own advocate. There is no one in this world who is going to fight for your child to come alive like you can.

Make God your partner in this fight--not any one doctor or medical professional. This doctor seemed so nice when I first met her, but ultimately she could have stolen my son's right to life away.

625. Understand That In Many Ways, This Journey Is One You Are Sometimes Going To Take Alon: Infertility can sometimes be a very lonely experience. Family and friends who love you dearly may not always be able to understand the depth of your pain.

Even your husband may not always understand your drive to have a baby. He might not always have the patience infertility demands. He will not always say and do the right thing.

While my husband wanted children as badly as I did, he sometimes lost patience with me and the whole process. Sometimes he thought I was too obsessive. Many times, I trudged on alone, because he was too tired and too angry to really be beside me through the ordeal. Other times, he was my knight in shining armor. We got along a lot better when I realized there were times I had to rely on myself and God, and not anyone else.

626. Find Places Where You Can Safely Pour Out Your Grief: Infertility can bring up a lot of grief, especially when things don't go right or are taking longer than you wish. You need places and people where you can pour out your grief in a safe, non-destructive way--not in a way that paralyzes or cripples you.

Do you have a friend who can listen to your intense grief and not lecture, criticize or try to get you to give up?

 Do you have a family member who is kind and can listen to your most intense feelings of anger, jealousy and grief, and not make you feel silly for your emotions?

 It is important that when you need it, you have a friend, a family member, or a group where you can voice your feelings without feeling judged.

This is not the time to confide in people who are downers on the subject of fertility, or somehow think it is okay to pop your balloon of hope. Surround yourself with people who believe in your body's ability to heal and who can see a positive outcome for your efforts.

Whether it is a friend at work who also went through infertility, a blogger, or your Mom, talk, vent, cry, brainstorm with those who are positive and who can give you a sense of 'I'm here for you' at this time.

Stay away from anyone who is negative or will say and do things that will rob you of your optimism or power.

Avoid those who find it hard to empower anyone except themselves. Don't share your sadness with those who might underhandedly steal your ability to see this all working out.

Confide in people who will be positive and upbeat about your getting pregnant.

I was fortunate enough to have a few people like that in my life.

My mother, for one, was my greatest cheerleader and helper.
She always told me she knew I could get pregnant and have a baby.

Leah, my dear sweet Leah, who also was my greatest cheerleader (you can have more than one).

Judy, my dear sweet Judy, who one day at work out of the blue looked at me and said, "I can see you with a little girl with cork screw curls." How did she know I would end up having a daughter with beautiful curls?

Or Peter, my dear beloved friend, that I phoned late one night when I was in despair, who declared without hesitation that I would get pregnant.

There were others too, but I will never forget the words of people who believed in a happy ending for me, when I could barely believe myself.

I cherish those friends and family members who said words that gave me hope instead of crushing my dream.

Beware of therapists or counselors who want to beat you down with "realism." At the infertility clinic I went to, there was a counselor who was like sheer poison to patients like me. In my darkest times, she said the most negative words to me and I have no idea why.

When you undergo infertility treatments, you need words of hope.

Your body needs to be told over and over and over again that it is strong enough, healthy enough, and capable of getting pregnant.

If you have a family member or friend who tends to be negative about the whole process, you need to ask them to please stop doing this. Once someone told me they thought God didn't want me to have children. I asked her to never, never say that to me again. Her words were stealing my hope, and I was feeling doubtful enough already. My body couldn't afford to listen to such negative predictions even for a minute.

You need to find people willing to hear your pain, see your tears, hear your screams of anger, and still say, "I think you will have a baby."

Understand that there are people in this world who, due to their own disappointing experiences, don't really believe people can do much to change their bad situations. They see going after a dream as a waste of time. Or maybe they are just jealous and unable to really wish good for anyone but themselves. They slyly discourage you, because they want to be the only one with a happy-ever-after story.

Others don't understand the power of choice, perseverance, and will.

They just don't get that today's no can be tomorrow's yes.

Some people have tried for dreams that never came true. They think they are doing you a favor by dousing you with realism, so you won't get disappointed. They are, of course, completely wrong.

Bottom line: confide only in positive, helpful, hopeful, people who aren't too afraid or too jealous or too sad themselves to see you have a win.

627. Understand the Power That Lies In Your Passionate Desire for Children: To endure all that is going to be asked of you, you need a mighty big motivator—and wanting a child passionately can be the motivation you need to get through this.

Your intense desire to be a mother will help you override the physical and emotional pain of infertility treatments. Your passionately wanting a child is an asset, not a liability. When the yearning and longing for a child feels intense and painful, remind yourself that it is this yearning and longing that will help see you through to your goal.
Feel the pride in knowing that your desire to love another human is that big, that consuming, that deep, and something you should respect yourself for.

628. Be Patient: When you are having trouble coping, remind yourself that getting healthy and restoring your fertility takes patience.

The body doesn't heal overnight. Once, after six months of weekly acupuncture treatments, I asked my acupuncturist if I was getting healthier. I expected glowing remarks about how all my effort was paying off. Instead, he answered, "A bit. You are still very weak." What? After all I had done? I was pretty discouraged.

I thought I was going to hear about all the progress I was making! Despite this not-so-encouraging diagnosis, I kept going to acupuncture weekly.

I had to be patient, whether I liked it or not. In time, I grew to understand that my body was changing and healing with every appointment, even if it was ever-so- slightly, and that continued effort would eventually see my body to a different and better place.

If you are making good choices for your body, keep on making these good choices. Eventually they will pay off, even if it takes all your patience to keep on track for the long haul.

629. Take Your Power, Acknowledge Your Power, Harness Your Power, Utilize Your Power: Never for a minute take a fatalistic approach to infertility. You can't control the outcome of your infertility treatments.

Nor are you at fault if this doesn't work out, but you do have some power in this situation.

Not total power. Not complete power, but you do have some power.

You have the power to pray. You have the power to stop letting foods, chemicals, toxic substances into your body that could weaken you. You have the power to believe in yourself. You have the power to eat well. You have power over how you use your words, and whether or not you will speak with positive belief or negative dread.

While you are not all powerful in this process, neither are you entirely helpless and powerless either. Whatever measure of power you have, grab hold of it and be aware of it.

630. During the Hard Times, Remember To Conjure Up Some Good Old-Fashioned Persistence: Remember the old saying: if at first you don't succeed, try, try again. This basic, bottom line way of thinking might mean the difference between having a baby and never having one.

Let yourself persist. Throw yourself over the bar and persevere, persevere, persevere. Don't see a no this month as a no forever. A no today does not mean a no tomorrow. I have a neighbor who did four IVFs—four! She was almost 45 years old, had only one working ovary and she miscarried a few times.

She had every reason to give up after three IVFS--but she didn't! Something inside her--call it faith, the ability to persevere, the ability to mourn the disappointments and heartbreaks and allow herself another try--and she continued on to number four.

Well, attempt number four turned out to be her winning try and she gave birth to a beautiful, healthy, lovely baby boy.

No one is going to lie and say persevering is easy. After you've had a few hard disappointments, it is hard to continue. But giving up can ultimately be the most disappointing turn of events of all. Keep trying if you can. Don't listen to people who try to make you quit.

Keep trying. Go for one more cycle. Don't listen to all the people who tell you to quit, that because it didn't work this month or this year or even for the past few years that obviously it is never going to work.
Ignore the people who say, "Can't you see that maybe you are not meant to...? Haven't you already tried this and that?" Shut them out of your brain.

One more time--and it may be the time your body is ready to be pregnant and deliver a baby. Do one more thing. Call one more person. Try another clinic. Persist, persist, persist. Bang on every door.

Read every book on health available, because one of those books may hold the answer for you. Get another physical and have your body checked completely. Do it again and again if you have to.
Don't be afraid to stomp your feet and scream, "I WANT A BABY AND I'M NOT GOING TO STOP UNTIL I HAVE ONE."

However, if you've come to a point where infertility is just too emotionally painful and you cannot hear one more no, consider the alternatives. Adoption is also having a real baby of your own, a beautiful option, and not one that precludes you from continuing to try for a biological child someday.

But if adoption is not something you feel ready to consider, don't give up trying to give birth to a baby. You might be inches away from your dream and not even know it.

Sometimes it is that one-more-try that can bring results.

631. Make The Process Of Infertility Treatments As Pleasurable As Possible: When I first learned that I would have to take shots every night to prepare for an IVF, I didn't think I was going to be able to handle it. But then I stumbled onto something that made the whole process easier and lighter: I had recently got a beautiful book of recipes from bed and breakfast inns. It was a sweet, pretty, cozy book, with recipes for things like blueberry muffins, apple butter and raspberry jam. I found that if I read a recipe from this book, while my husband gave me my shots, the whole thing was a lot more bearable.

This lovely book had a beautiful white and blue cover. Just looking it would calm me down.

So instead of looking at the needle about to be jabbed in my leg, I put my eyes on this romantic little cookbook, and I was whisked away to quaint inns across the country, visions of blueberry this-or-that dancing in my head.

You, also, can find ways to make the most difficult moments in your treatment bearable.

Listen to great music while driving to the infertility clinic.

Get to know the nurses and other medical staff at the clinic, and bring them flowers occasionally--brightening up their day can give you a boost too.

632. Stop The 'I Should Have' or 'I Shouldn't Have' Talk: Infertility is not your fault. Stop blaming yourself, with thoughts like, 'I should have had children sooner' or 'I shouldn't have done this or that.' This is not your fault. For some reason, infertility seems to be an illness where women like to blame themselves.

633. Harness the Power of Positive Words When The Nurse Calls With Disappointing News: You need to be aware of the self-talk that occurs within you when a cycle doesn't work out. When you hear a 'no', do you say to yourself, 'this will never work out for me.'

Be very watchful of the words you use, especially when you hit a bump in the road. Your body listens to the conversations you have with yourself and it follows suit.

If you say things like, "I probably won't ever get pregnant" well, if you have an obedient body, it might just live up (or down) to your expectations. After you get off the phone with a nurse who has devastating news, before you start crying, repeat these words: tomorrow it will all work out for me, tomorrow it will all work out for me, tomorrow it will all work out for me.

Use your words to propel you towards what you want.

Let words come out of your mouth that will help create a positive, healthy vibration within you.

Even in your most difficult moments, speak of getting pregnant as if it already happened. Let your words stamp on you a definite 'yes, my body will physically manifest a baby soon.'

If a cycle didn't work out, say to yourself: my body is getting more and more fertile every day. Or 'my baby is on their way to me.'

Never let yourself say words that carry a defeated, sad prediction for yourself.

Keep repeating, "I will get pregnant and have a baby...I will get pregnant and have a baby...I will get pregnant and have a baby" regardless of how disappointed and sad you are feeling.

634. Coping With the Unfairness of It All: Is it fair that you should have to suffer with infertility, when other women seem to get pregnant without barely trying? Is it fair that you are invited to yet another baby shower for the lady down the street who already has two adorable kids? No, it isn't fair at all. Do you have a right to feel sorry for yourself? Yes, you definitely do. But just because something is not fair doesn't mean that ultimately you can't get what came easily to someone else. Maybe your road is harder and longer than some other women, but you can reach the same destination as much as a person who got pregnant without trying.

635. Give Yourself A Break and Get Away: If you are feeling overwhelmed, consider a vacation, a day trip or a weekend away. It could be something simple, like a visit to a lake less than an hour from your house, a trip to the beach, an afternoon at a local park or museum. A change in environment can sometimes give you the break you need.

Take some time to discover places within a 30 minute drive that can give you that same feeling of rest, peace, and escape. A change of environment might be exactly what you need.

636. Take Daily Mini-Vacations: Maybe you can't get away on a vacation right now—but you can enjoy daily mini-vacations. Start by listing three places within 15 minutes of your home that you can enjoy on a daily or weekly basis.

Some examples include:

a favorite park
a walking trail
a relaxing bookstore
a fun and interesting store
a friend's home where you feel loved and accepted
a home of a wonderful relative
a place of worship
a restaurant within your budget
a bowling alley
a coffeehouse
a farm or farmstand
a lake
a pond
a walking trail
a college campus
a pool
a library
a newspaper stand
an animal rescue center (lots of little kittens put a smile on my face!)
an outdoor garden
a museum with outdoor benches

637. Read and Flood your Mind with Hopeful, Positive, Miracle Stories: Go to a bookstore or library and find hopeful, inspirational stories that lift your spirits. Read uplifting passages from the Bible. Read the life stories of people who overcame almost impossible adversities. Read stories in the Bible of people like Hannah and Sarah. There is a lot of information out there that is negative, discouraging and cynical. Avoid this information at all costs. Avoid reading information on infertility that is loaded with discouraging statistics.

Avoid any form of disaster reading. Refuse to take in information that sours your spirit and leaves you feeling hopeless. If ever in your life there was a time to feed yourself as much optimism and hope as possible, it is now. Read personal growth books that uplift, encourage, and bring you to a place of joy. I typed up passages from the Bible and positive messages from various books and I read them daily.

638. Press Your Happy Buttons—A lot!!: To keep going, you need to press your 'happy buttons' as often as possible. A happy button can be rereading a much loved book, hanging a picture in your home that brings you joy, or enjoying a dinner out at a restaurant you love. You need to pursue putting your body into a state of joy as much as possible--because it is in this state that healing and conception has a better chance of taking place.

639. Don't Listen To Anyone Who Blames You For Your Infertility: If someone tries to criticize you or blame you for your infertility, walk away, ignore them, refuse to listen. If someone says: 'you are just too uptight' or you are having trouble getting pregnant because you are..." Say: thanks, but no thanks. Here's an alert: millions of women who are uptight, nervous and stressed get pregnant every day.

Fertility is a complicated medical condition and no one is to blame. The body sometimes does what it is suppose to do and sometimes it doesn't. But...(and here's the but)...just because the body isn't doing what it is suppose to do today doesn't mean it won't make a switch and do exactly what it is suppose to do tomorrow.

So tell any well-meaning, but oh-so-annoying-people, that IT IS NOT YOUR FAULT and walk away. You don't have time to listen to this garbage.

640. Treat and Alleviate Depression: Doctors have found that infertile women can boost their odds of getting pregnant by alleviating their depression. However, the catch-22 is: being infertile can cause depression, so how do you treat depression while battling infertility that can cause depression?

• Increase your intake of folic acid. Researchers have found that blood levels among those with depression had much lower levels of folate (folic acid).

• Take a high-quality B-complex. The B vitamins have been shown to help reduce depression.

• Find out if you have an iron deficiency. Depression is often a symptom of chronic iron deficiency.

• Take a high-quality calcium/magnesium supplement.

• Lack of the mineral zinc is linked to depression. Low levels of zinc in the body have been shown to result in paranoia and fearfulness.

• Include omega-3s and foods rich in omega-3s in your diet more often.

• Increase your social support. Join a support group, a neighborhood book club, or attend a weekly meeting with those you have something in common with. Positive social support can do much to alleviate depression.

• Learn how to deep breath.

• Try to include in your daily schedule time with supportive people, friends and family; a mild form of exercise, time outdoors, and time helping others in some way, such as writing a card to a sick friend, sewing a blanket for a children's hospital, or dropping off some baked goods for a friend.

• Restructure how you talk to yourself—remember: positive words, positive words, positive words.

You deserve an internal best friend who speaks kindly to you, not an internal enemy that is always badgering you.

• Keep your blood sugar levels stable by eating several times a day and avoid white flour and sugary foods.

• Tell yourself 'I love you" several times a day. Whenever you start to feel sad or hopeless, say, "I love you" to yourself.

641. How To Respond To Some of the Rude Comments You May Hear Along the Way from Family and Friends: This is not to be misinterpreted as an exercise in dumping family or friends, because people are not perfect and we should not expect them to be, and there are people in our lives, as unpleasant as they may be, that we simply need to forgive, stay connected to and be around. Despite their flaws, we owe them something. That being said, as you walk this journey, you need to be ready for some of the stupid, rude and totally insensitive comments you are going to hear. Sometimes, people you love will say really dumb things. Other times, it could be a stranger who zaps you with a statement that leaves you breathless and feeling punched in the gut.

Here are a few of the stupid, rude, thoughtless and COMPLETELY FALSE comments you may have to deal with, and how best to respond:

642. "Maybe you weren't meant to have a baby": Yes, you were meant to have a baby. Yes, you were. Millions of women have babies whether they want them or not, whether they will be good mothers or not, so why shouldn't you have a baby? In fact, there is NOT ONE REASON IN THIS UNIVERSE why you should not have a baby.

This person is either jealous of you or just likes to pop the balloon of hope. People who mouth off a comment like this mistakenly feel they have some sort of moral authority. Ignore them. They are wrong. Completely and utterly wrong.

643. "Aren't you a little too old to be trying for a baby?": Whoever got the idea that a young mother is better than an older mother has not seen the millions of mothers in their 40s and even 50s who mother with great patience, love, insight, wisdom and kindness.

This person obviously doesn't understand that with age comes maturity and wisdom. Someone who makes a comment like this may be focusing on the energy level of children, forgetting that even most 25 year old mothers are not out playing baseball with their kids everyday.

Whoever throws out a comment about age is ignorant of the fact that a woman of any age who is ready and able to love a child, and who is brave and strong enough to endure infertility, is more prepared, capable and ready to mother than almost anyone. A good mother is a good mother, whether she is 21, 31, 41, 51 or beyond.

644. "Why don't you just adopt?": A person who says this perhaps does not understand or is not sensitive to the desire to have biological children. Maybe they don't have children, so to them, what difference does it make how you get a child. Or they have children and it came so easily and naturally, that they don't see it as a privilege or any big deal.

Here's the thing: adoption is a wonderful opportunity for those who are ready and willing to embrace it. However, if this is not the path you desire, DO NOT FEEL GUILTY!!!!! You have every right to a biological child, and even if your desire for a biological child isn't coming easily— IT DOESN'T MEAN YOU WON'T HAVE ONE EVENTUALLY. This type of comment throws guilt in a direction it should not be thrown. Adoption is something that a person should do only if they passionately want to, not because they feel guilted into doing it. You have a right to want a biological child, and a right to take advantage of whatever is medically available to make that happen. No one has the right to make you feel guilty about this, and or rob you of a natural right.

645. "Don't worry! Just relax and it will happen": This comment often comes with all the best intentions. Perhaps this person feels sympathy for you, but doesn't know what to say to express themselves.

Maybe they don't know much about infertility and are not educated on how the reproductive system works.

Maybe they want to comfort you, and this is their attempt to do so. Maybe they mistakenly believe that by saying this, you will relax a bit and get pregnant. When you get this type of advice, you need to remember that millions of women get pregnant every day under all kinds of conditions, including stress, war, famine and other horrific environments that are definitely not relaxing.

It is very unlikely that as you go through infertility you are always going to feel blissed-out and relaxed—and for that, you should not feel guilty.

"Maybe its for the best. Maybe you couldn't handle it"

This comment often comes from either someone who has children and really doesn't enjoy being a mother, and deep down feels they were handed something they couldn't handle, or the person is the competitive type who likes to one-up others and takes odd pleasure in put downs.

When you get this type of comment, remind yourself that you are going to be a great mother. Just because no one has seen you in action yet, doesn't mean you are not going to be the best mother around.

Your friends and family have not seen your maternal side in action yet. Maybe at this point, they are unable to envision the mother you are going to be. Maybe they are so focused on lifestyle choices, personality traits, and attitudes that serve you well now that they can't see the maternal potential inside you. But just wait—someday they will stand back in awe at the amazing mother you are.

If you desire to love a child, then you will find ways to raise your child in safety and love, whether you have any experience caring for a child or not.

If someone doesn't see your potential to do that, well, they are clueless as to who you really are.

Hold tight to the vision you have of yourself as a mother regardless of how others see you—other people can often only see what is right in front of their eyes and do not have the insight to see the maternal flower inside of you waiting and ready to bloom.

646. "Having children at your age is risky. They might be born with a disability or special need": This comment most likely comes from a person who likely always sees the glass half full, lives their life in fear, and does not embrace risk. They also like spreading their gloom around, perhaps because they see trouble lurking around the corner, instead of opportunity and hope.

Here's a little thing someone who makes a comment like this doesn't realize: any child can be born with a disability and age doesn't have as much to do with it as we like to think. Having a child at any age, even for teenagers, comes with some risks. Good prenatal care and nutrition can do much to eliminate the risks. Be brave and step forward, and don't let those who lack courage stop you.

Their warnings are not warnings that will protect you in any way. In fact, their warnings are actually vicious thieves who could rob you of what you want most. Feel sorry for anyone who says this to you: life is probably a bit too scary for them to ever enjoy.

647. "I'm the opposite. All my husband had to do is walk by me and I got pregnant": Wow, this person really likes to feel better than others and gets a real kick out of a chance to self-promote how great they are. Tisk, tisk, tisk, didn't their mother teach them better than this?

Maybe you should just congratulate them and say something like, 'wow, you are so much better than me. I wish I was like you" because bottom line is that is exactly what they want to hear.

Just remember: some women get pregnant easily and some don't—and someday, when you are snuggling with your beautiful baby, it won't really matter how you got to your moment and how they got to their moments, because you will be enjoying the same prize.

It isn't fair, of course, that their road may have been a lot easier than yours—but ultimately, you can have exactly what they have and more. Plus, you'll always have your good manners that they obviously lack.

648. 'Maybe God doesn't want you to have a baby': In my opinion, whoever dares say this to you is stepping on sacred ground. Ask them: when did God give you the right to speak for Him? Since when do they get to speak God's intentions for you? According to the Bible, God loves us and wants great things for us. God is love—and love never denies, but gives. This person really has no understanding of God's true personality. Perhaps they should sit down and read the Bible closely. God is complete goodness and love—not some punishing father ready to deny us. If they see God this way, perhaps they need to get to know Him better. It is rude, presumptuous and ignorant to speak for God or to assume that a physical condition like infertility is the result of God's withholding something from one of His earthly children.

Would they say to a person with cancer, "this is God's will for you." Probably not—because we look at other diseases as physical problems that deserve treatment. So why is infertility a disease that is viewed differently?

Ignore this person and remind yourself of the scripture at 1 John 4:8, "God is love" and spend some time thinking about how someone who is pure love gives and provides, not takes away and denies.

If this statement is ever thrown at you, immediately begin repeating: God is love, God is love, God is love, over and over again.

649. "Didn't you try this before and it didn't work out?": Yup, and trying again is what winners do so they ultimately get what they want. A person who might not like to repeat their efforts without immediate reward—also known as lazy—might come up with this one. Again, ignore and move on. They don't know what they are talking about.

650. "I went through infertility treatments and they didn't work": Of course, sympathize and feel badly for this person, but remember: their journey doesn't have to be your journey. Their experience doesn't have to be your experience. Their outcome is not going to be your outcome.

Just because it hasn't worked out for them yet doesn't mean it isn't going to work out for you. Different people, different choices, different results. They are not hopeless and either are you.

Whether or not they ever have a baby doesn't mean you do not have the right to get the children you want. Don't bother arguing with that person or trying to convince them that your path will be different than theirs. Be kind and walk away. New treatments, new medications, and new ways of healing from infertility are being offered everyday.

And remember: you have every right to have this work out—even it didn't work out for someone else.

651. "Aren't infertility treatments dangerous? I hear the medications can cause this or that": Well, doesn't everything have a little bit of danger in it? It takes courage and the ability to risk-take to go after anything in this world. If you want a baby, than any obstacle is worth climbing over to get it. Danger/smanger/ignore and move on.

652. "If I were you, I wouldn't get so worked up about this": Well, obviously, they are not you. Maybe this person never really wanted anything that badly. Or maybe they are just super insensitive to other people's pain. Whatever the reason for such a comment, it shows a lack of insight—infertility is very much a reason to be worked up. This passion will also make you a great mother someday.

653. "You've already been through so much. If I were you, I'd give up": Well, I'll say it again--they are not you—you are stronger, braver and able to walk through fire to get what you want. Maybe they just don't have the guts you have. Maybe they already have what they want, or they don't want anything that badly, that seeing you make so much effort is unnerving to them. Don't listen. Be proud that you can continue on despite the difficulty involved.

How To Not Let Infertility Ruin Your Marriage

654. Infertility can be rough on a marriage. From the day you start infertility treatments, it will be best if you let go of the idea that your husband will always be able to fully understand and care for all the emotions you will experience in the quest to have a baby.

Let go of the idea that he will always say the right thing. Abandon the hope that he will always know exactly how to comfort you.

As much as my husband wanted children, he did not always understand my raw anguish or single-minded drive. Looking back, I shouldn't have expected him to understand all my emotions. It was a waste of time and energy I needed to put into my healing.

What I didn't understand was that, while my husband's desire to have children was strong, he manifested it differently than I did.

Sometimes I became enraged when I felt he was being a bit too clinical about the whole experience.

Don't try to get your husband to express his desire for a baby in the exact same way you do. It is pointless. Your husband cannot be the focus of your frustration right now.

Doing things to make your body healthier is where your energy needs to be, not in fighting with your husband over his perceived insensitivities.

Some husbands are just not able to fully grasp the intense passion, fervor and sometimes obsession a woman can feel over having a baby.

If your husband does understand, you are very fortunate.

If not, that's okay too.

Just remember--this journey isn't about him--it is about bringing the baby of your dreams to life. Wasting time arguing with him or expecting him to totally relate to your feelings is, well, a waste of time.

As much as you need his support right now, you need to empower yourself and find your strength within. If you can, build a network of support outside of your marriage, so that he won't be your exclusive source of comfort.

Don't expect him to rescue you from the pain and work involved in infertility treatments. Don't expect him to mother you, nurse you, or completely get what this means to you.

Do expect he may say exactly what you don't want him to say at exactly the wrong time.

Many husbands end up becoming true heroes to their wives during infertility treatments, but even those who rise to the challenge can sometimes disappoint--not because they are insensitive or uncaring, but simply because they might be tired, cranky, or feeling intense emotions of their own.

Infertility is tiring and sometimes people run out of steam.

For the times when perhaps he is insensitive, forgive him and let it go. Don't waste time moping and groaning about how he doesn't get it.

Remember: your husband cannot save you from the pain of this ordeal, or erase the frustration and rage you sometimes are going to feel.

Don't make trying to get him to understand your feelings your mission-- you will be wasting precious time and emotional resources. Don't expect him to be driven in exactly the same way you are, although some men are.

Most likely all this infertility stuff is going to stress out your relationship, and you can't take too seriously anything you feel about each other at this time. The goal is to give birth to your baby, not make your husband feel the same maternal longing you feel. Infertility treatments are extremely grueling work, and your husband may get impatient with the whole ordeal. Or you may be one of the fortunate ones, and have a husband as dedicated and motivated as you are.

My husband and I fought a lot during our infertility treatments, especially the first time. The stress was sometimes too much for us to handle. We often turned on each another. I'm not sure what would have prevented this. I needed him to be more tender and he needed me to be more understanding. We both needed to be a lot kinder to each other.

At my lowest points, I desperately wanted him to say some magic words that would make me feel better, and frankly, I was enraged when he didn't seem to have those magic words.

Looking back, most of our fights were wasted energy--just a place and a distraction to put all our anger and sadness over the situation.

I wish I had used that time more wisely. The second time around, I focused more on my battle to get healthy, instead of looking to my husband to rescue me. Issues with my husband faded into the background once I had my priorities straight, although in my darkest times, my darling, sweet, strong husband was my greatest ally, and ultimately, he worked just as hard as I did through the process. For his perseverance, I am forever grateful.

Once, after an IVF cycle didn't work out, my husband said he needed to go for a drive alone to deal with the pain. Somehow, knowing he hurt as much as I did helped me not feel so alone.

While my husband and I did turn on each other at times, especially when we were sad, ultimately he was my hero.

After a laparoscopy procedure when I woke up in excruciating pain, it was my husband who kneeled by my bed, rubbed my feet and did everything in his power to ease my pain. So as hard as infertility can be on a marriage, it can also bring you closer than you were before.

Your husband may support you in ways you never even imagined. Just don't be disappointed when he can't.

There are things, however, you can do to help him through this journey.

First, keep the happy chemicals in his brain going, and at the same time, enhance his sperm quality, with zinc, Vitamin C, Vitamin E, folic acid, magnesium, omega-3, lots of greens, vegetables, pumpkin seeds, oysters, selenium and L-Carnitine. Take relaxing walks together. Remember to say thank you and show appreciation for those times when he does help you in exactly the way you need.

As hard as it is, try to do some fun things together during this time. Maybe try golf or fishing or some other relaxing, non-demanding sport, like sand castle building or bird watching. Take a break, sometimes, and do something completely romantic. Always remember to kiss and make-up when times get tough.

The goal is not to turn on each other during this stressful time, and not to let unrealistic expectations about what your husband is suppose to do or feel cause problems in your marriage.

 Hopefully, you will receive the support you need from your husband. When you don't, let it go and focus on your goal.

655. **How To Choose The Right Doctor:** Don't underestimate the importance of having a good doctor, and don't ever be naive about the damage the wrong doctor can do. Frankly, the wrong doctor can steal your chance of having a baby and the family you dream of.

Start by researching infertility clinics in your area. You want to choose a clinic with high success rates and an esteemed reputation. You want a doctor who is a fertility specialist and affiliated with a highly reputable fertility clinic with a high success rate.

A gynecologist may not have as much experience as a specialist who focuses exclusively on infertility. They may also lack the resources and access to the latest reproductive technologies.

Research the success rates of various clinics within 30 minutes to an hour from your home. When choosing a clinic, weigh carefully the travel time and route to the clinic. You will be going to the clinic a lot, sometimes every day for weeks. If travel is no consideration, go to the best clinic within an hour from you.

When choosing a clinic, make sure they have a wide range of fertility treatments available and are familiar with the latest technologies. If you have choices, try to select a clinic that makes you feel comfortable, doesn't stress you out, and who can offer you the best and most choices. If you know others dealing with infertility, ask for their opinions and experiences at different clinics with different doctors.

I found the doctor who helped me become pregnant with my son through a neighbor he also helped conceive and give birth to her son.

It is important that you select a doctor you feel comfortable with and who answers your questions. If a doctor refuses to answer your questions or seems to dismiss your questions, this may not be the doctor to select.

If they almost come off as disrespectful and arrogant, than perhaps then you need to ask yourself: will they listen if I request a certain test or change in medications? Or will they ignore my requests?

Ideally, you want a doctor who listens to your recommendations and orders whatever tests and medications you request.

A doctor who doesn't put the time into finding solutions for you may not be the right doctor.

While physicians in the infertility industry are very busy and it is not realistic to expect excessive emotional support, you should be able to expect one who listens and pays attention to your requests, is determined to help you, and is willing to try new procedures and medications. Some fertility doctors may seem cold because they have large caseloads.

Occasionally, doctors with high success rates can sometimes have a hidden agenda in trying to get you to quit the attempt for a biological child. Before following the recommendations of a doctor, always consider where their motive for your course of treatment might be coming from.

If you are of an advanced age, every time you do an IUI or an IVF and it fails, their success rates for live births are lowered, and thus it is in their best interests to persuade you to try an alternative method that precludes the attempt at a biological child so their statistics remain high. Could your continuing to pursue the goal of having biological children lower their live birth rate statistics? Is this a doctor more concerned with their stats than with helping you achieve your goal? For those who can maintain high live birth statistics, it means higher rankings and more customers.

Also stay alert to how long you are kept on a medication, especially if it is not working. Is your doctor keeping track of your progress and alert to when a change in medication is needed? If you have suffered miscarriages, did your doctor prescribe or suggest progesterone for future pregnancies? Are they making an attempt to give you what you need so you don't miscarry again?

Do not stay with a doctor who is not producing results for you, or at least trying to find what is going to work for you. If your doctor stays with the same protacol repeatedly, despite no success, it might be time to get another doctor.
Or at least see if your doctor is willing to sit down and reevaluate your treatment plan.

It is important that you don't get stuck trusting just one medical professional to the point that you waste years with someone who isn't getting results for you, or is just on the wrong track altogether. Be open to finding a new doctor, even one within the clinic you go to, when if time has passed and there is no progress or results.

You need a doctor willing to switch gears, and try different tactics to get you pregnant. You want a doctor who is willing to acknowledge when it is time to try something new in your treatment.

You don't need a doctor so tied up in ego, so stuck on one way of doing things, that they don't venture out and try every available medicine and procedure out there. You want a doctor who will investigate why things are not working out for you.

If you strongly feel you need certain tests and your doctor refuses to do them, by all means find a new doctor. If you ask for a change in medication and that request is ignored, it is time to find another doctor.

After an IVF that failed, I went to my doctor with a list of questions and a request for a new medication I had read about and researched that seemed like it would help me.

This doctor refused to answer even one of my questions, told me my eggs were bottom of the barrel and I should quit trying, wanted to give me an ovarian reserve test to determine whether my fertility was over, and would not even consider trying the new medication.

I went home, called the clinic, and changed doctors immediately, thanks to some very wise advice from my mother.

I then chose a doctor within the clinic that my neighbor had. He had helped her become pregnant with her beautiful son. What a change! My new doctor answered every one of my questions and immediately agreed that this new medication was one that he would definitely try and was considering before I even suggested it.

Two months later, I was pregnant with my son, who I gave birth to nine months later.

That other doctor was completely wrong. If I had listened to her, I probably would have given up. If I had taken that ovarian reserve test, and somehow it showed my ovarian reserve to be low, my insurance company may have then denied my right to fertility treatments. Why did she want to put me in such a position that my treatments would no longer be covered and I could not afford to pay them out of pocket. Perhaps she had too many patients and didn't have time for a patient like me. Maybe she got the ranking of 'best in' my area because she pushed patients towards using egg donors rather than their own eggs because with younger eggs comes a higher chance of live births, thus falsely elevating her success rate. When patients of advanced age use their own eggs, the risk of failure is higher, and she did not want the failed IVFs that would lower her success rate.

Do you see how dangerous listening to the wrong doctor can be?

The first doctor didn't really care about me or the outcome of my treatments. She simply didn't want to be bothered with me anymore. She didn't think my desire for a biological child was worth one more try.

The next doctor was accommodating, hard working and willing to try a new treatment plan.

As I said before, the wrong doctor can steal your chance to have a baby, while the right doctor can play a significant role in making your dream happen.

Make sure the doctor you choose is organized. Does your doctor seem scattered, like they are more concerned with publishing in medical journals than actually practicing medicine?

Do they seem hassled, like they have taken on too many patients and cannot handle the workload? If so, they may make poor decisions when it comes to your care.

The doctor I mentioned above was named one of the best in my region by a well-respected magazine, but she mistakenly diagnosed me as having fibroids. I underwent a procedure to remove them, but it turned out I did not have fibroids at all. She never apologized for the unnecessary pain and time wasted on this operation that she caused me. Because of this operation, my fertility treatments were delayed for months.

If you have friends who also are being treated for infertility, or were treated successfully, ask for their recommendations and feedback. But take note: while you can listen to suggestions, you need to follow your own gut feelings. A doctor might be right for one person, but not another. At the same time, if you have a friend you share a lot in common with, and they found success with a certain doctor, you might want to schedule a 'getting to know you' meeting with their doctor and see for yourself. Note how your body feels when you are with this doctor—do you leave feeling agitated or calm? Confident or unsure of yourself? Never overlook or deny nagging feelings of doubt.

How do you know you chose the wrong doctor?

You know you have the wrong doctor when the doctor does not explore every possible reason for your infertility, refuses to listen to your ideas, does not answer your questions, and does not try new medications and treatments to help you get pregnant.

The wrong doctor never admits when they are wrong, and they stubbornly stay tethered to a plan that doesn't work. The wrong doctor is not knowledgeable on all the reasons you may be infertile and is not aware of all the new medications available.

The wrong doctor is more concerned with their statistics than in trying to help you. The wrong doctor will try to push you in a direction you may not want to go. The wrong doctor will take away your hope.

Never take the word of one doctor as if they were God.

Even if you really like your doctor and have a wonderful relationship, be sure to question, analyze and investigate the course of treatment they give you.

You may be taking the word or accepting the decisions of one doctor who may be on the wrong track, or who might not have your best interests in mind, or might be a bit lazy, or have too many patients, or who may simply be too arrogant to realize a change in your treatment is needed. Or simply—your doctor might be great, but is still failing to get you on the right medication or treatment plan.

If you are not getting pregnant, and it has been a long time, try a new doctor, get a second opinion, don't stay tethered to any one doctor or clinic if you don't see results or they are not listening to your concerns. Even if you find a doctor you like, if they do not produce results for you after a certain amount of time, go and get another opinion. This is not the time for you to be stuck on one doctor to the point that you don't aggressively pursue every test, medication and treatment that will get you pregnant.

Initially, I liked that doctor who led me down the wrong path. She was comforting during certain procedures and had a likeable personality. But ultimately, she was a danger to my fertility. That's why when it comes to choosing and staying with a doctor, keep your eyes open and keep close track of your progress.

Here are some common mistakes those suffering with infertility often encounter:

656. Waiting too long to get help: Stop listening to those people who tell you to simply relax and it will happen. Relaxing does help, but it is not the only solution. If you've been trying to get pregnant for awhile and it is not happening, see an infertility specialist immediately.

657. undergoing infertility treatments, never forget the old saying, "if at first you don't succeed, try, try again." Even if you have done several cycles, if you feel you can cope and want to continue, let yourself try again. Don't listen to those who say, 'you've tried X number of times and if it hasn't work yet it isn't going to.' The next try could be the one that works.

658. Not seeing the correlation between poor eating habits, and infertility: Don't get tricked into believing that you can eat any way you want and it won't impact your fertility. Everything you consume impacts your fertility—and it your responsibility to start getting this part of your life right.

659. Not strengthening every part of your body, from your liver, to your kidney to your adrenal glands: You know various ways to detoxify and strengthen your organs—so go ahead and do it.

660. Not participating in your own healing process and thinking it is someone else's responsibility: Your doctor and the infertility clinic can provide you with a treatment plan and medications to help you get pregnant, but the rest of the healing is up to you.

661. Not Trying To Discover The Root Cause of Your Infertility: Even if your doctor diagnoses you with 'unexplained infertility' the bottom line is there is a reason you are not getting pregnant—one that perhaps is so subtle that the clinics have no precise test that can diagnose it.

That is where it is in your best interests to seek out holistic and alternative medicine to address the subtle reasons your body is not conceiving naturally.

662. **How to Cope With Stress:** You've heard it a million times before. Now you will hear it again: stress is a huge enemy of your fertility. Stress weakens your body, impacts your hormones, and could be what is standing between you and your future children.

Stress makes your body a less welcoming and hospitable place. Some doctors believe that stress plays a role in 20 to 30 percent of all infertility cases.

The reason stress is so dangerous to your fertility is it elevates hormones like cortisol and epinephrine, which inhibit the body's main sex hormone gonadotropin releasing hormone (GnRH).

Stress inhibits the release of reproductive hormones. GnRH is responsible for the pituitary gland's release of luteinizing hormones and follicle-stimulating hormones.

Stress disrupts hormone communication between your brain, pituitary and ovaries, thus interfering with the maturation of the egg and ovulation process.

Stress can also kick the body into a fight or flight response that makes it difficult for the body to feel safe enough to get pregnant.

However, it should be noted that all around the world, lots of women are very stressed and get pregnant anyways. Stress is part of life, and yes, you will feel stressed sometimes during this process. I am not in any way saying: 'relax you will get pregnant' because there are many underlying, hard to detect physical reasons pregnancy is not occurring.

It is disrespectful to suggest that a person going through infertility treatments would somehow not feel stressed.

Of course you are going to be stressed! How could you not? So, don't feel guilty if sometimes you feel stressed.

However, you deserve to stack the odds in your favor, and do whatever you can to reduce the stress hormones in your body.

Here are some suggestions:

663. Take Some Time to Analyze Exactly What in Your Life Stresses You: For a few days, write down every time you feel stressed. What caused you to feel stressed? Where were you? Who were you with? What was happening that made you feel this way? Then, ask yourself: are these stressors something I can change?

Write down ways you can change the stress triggers in your life. If these stressors are not factors you can change, ask yourself: can I change my attitude or how I talk to myself about these stressors so I do not get as upset next time?

The goal is to identify your stressors and find ways to change your circumstances so these triggers are no longer in your life. Or, if you cannot change the stressful situations in your life, can you change the way you react, think, talk to yourself about, and cope with these stressors?

An example: you realize that your daily commute to work is very stressful. Is there an alternative route you could take? A co-worker you could drive in with? A form of public transportation that would be more relaxing? A favorite CD or book you could play while you drive to help change your mood and what you think about as you drive? Would your employer be open to a change in work schedule that might lessen the traffic you encounter? Are there any opportunities for jobs closer to home or work-from-home days? What could you say to yourself during your commute that you can change? Start thinking of ways to address the situations that bring up feelings of stress in your life.

664. Repeat Positive Sayings and Positive Words: If you find you get stressed around a certain person or at a certain time of day, choose a saying or mantra that you can repeat over and over to yourself that will help calm you down.

Sayings that might help include:

Let go and let God
With God all things are possible
Everything will be all right
Been there, done that, all will turn out well
Breathe, breathe, breathe
Time for my bath
This too shall pass
Keep calm and carry on
Keep calm and love
I don't worry, I be happy
I s-m-i-l-e
I don't have to be perfect
I choose happy
I choose good
The sun is shining on me
Right now, a batch of warm chocolate chips cookies are coming out of the oven
I breathe peace
I breathe love
Stay calm—it will be all right
Inch by inch, life's a cinch
One bite at a time
Relax, God is in charge
God loves me and will take care of me
Love is here right now
It will be okay
I did good
Peace is mine
I will conquer

I smile with joy
My happy heart is light
Love is here, love is mine, love is everywhere
Courage is mine
My heart is smiling
Hope arrived!
I stand by you
Life is beautiful
Once upon a time there was a princess named <u>your name here</u>
I am happy
I feel wonderful
I am love

Choose a mantra that elicits positive feelings within you. For example, if you relax when you hear the word 'chocolate' or 'joy' create a saying you can repeat each day around those words, such as 'I have chocolate covered joy."

665. Put Yourself In Situations Or Around People That Make You Feel Safe: Feelings of danger often bring up stress in the body. Do whatever you can to increase your feelings of safety at this time. If you feel safe wrapped in a certain blanket drinking tea, make that part of your daily routine. If hearing your mother's voice or cuddling with your cat make you feel safe, do those things more often. Feeling safe helps us relax. If you can, avoid situations where you feel you are in danger.

666. Spend Ten Minutes Every Morning and Every Night Doing Deep Breathing Exercises: Inhale for a count of four, exhale for a count of four. Or, put one hand on your chest, one on your belly, and deep breath through your nose. Try alternate nostril breathing, where you hold the right thumb over your right nostril and inhale deeply. At the peak of inhalation, close off the left nostril and exhale through the right nostril. You can also try a long, slow inhale, and then a quick, powerful exhale from the lower belly.

667. Start Swimming: Swim indoors, outdoors, at a health club, a gym, in the ocean, a lake, or a river. Swimming was a big stress reliever for me. I always come out of the water feeling better than when I go in.

Swimming relaxes the body because it requires alternating stretch and relaxation of sketal muscles, while simultaneously deep-breathing in a rhythmic pattern. A note here: swimming might be best before you do an IVF or IUI cycle in order to relax the body. After an IVF treatment, it might be best to stop all exercises that are too extreme or harsh on the body, and this could include swimming.

668. Write Poetry: Write a poem, read uplifting poetry or choose an author and read all their poetry, either to yourself, aloud or start a poetry reading group. Some great poets include Walt Whitman, Maya Angelou, Robert Frost, Langston Hughes, Elizabeth Barrett Browning, William Shakespeare, Robert Browning, Henry Wadsworth Longfellow.

669. Get Your Hands Dirty: That's right—research has shown that touching dirt relieves stress. Plant some flowers, grow a potted herb garden, dig up some weeds, plant vegetables, flowers, grass. Just put your hands in the dirt and enjoy.

670. Spend More Time in Nature: Many studies have been done on the healing effects of green space on reducing stress and tension. The natural world offers some of the best relaxers available. Levels of serotonin, a neurotransmitter that regulates our moods, rise when we are outside in nature. Make it a goal to be outside at least 15 to 30 minutes a day, even if it just means sitting on the front steps of your apartment or in your driveway.

Smell nature, stare at nature, sit in nature, and be in the moment with nature. Go barefoot. When you are unable to get outdoors, take some pictures of natural scenes and display them in your home or workplace, so you can enjoy the peaceful serene feeling being in nature can bring.

Take daily walks in a park. Sit under a tree. Put your hands in the dirt and garden. Sit on your front lawn and take in the sunshine. Bring a sketchpad to a park and draw. Feed the birds, the deers, the seagulls, the turkeys. Hike a local trail every morning. Choose a spot and stare at a tree. Sit on the beach. Lay down in the grass. Have a picnic at a local lake. Swing on some swings. Read a book outside. Grow some grass in a pot and sniff it. Touch a tree. Pick up some pine needles, or sticks.

671. Bring Flowers Into Your Life: Buy yourself flowers weekly. Various studies have shown that we feel less negative and more energized when we are around flowers. At some local supermarkets, bouquets of flowers can often be enjoyed for $5 or less. Put flowers in a visible place where you can see and enjoy them, such as by your bed, on the kitchen table, or on your desk at work.

672. Hum Your Way to a Baby: Music can be a powerful tool in lifting our moods and relaxing our bodies. Music has been used as a healing tool for thousands of years, and it can be a healing therapy for you too. Research has shown that music sets off a neurological chain in the body that alleviates stress and induces relaxation.

As you undergo infertility treatments, begin using music as a way to relieve stress and elicit feelings of joy and hope. Commit to bringing more music into your life. Buy and play music from happy times in your life. Play music that lifts you up or relaxes you. Avoid sad, depressing music that makes you melancholy or reminds you of sad events in your life. Play Broadway show tunes, inspirational music, music that you love to dance to. Play whatever type of music calms you and helps you feel happy. Try some classical music. Play Italian love songs at dinner.

Keep a stereo in your living room or kitchen, and listen to music while cooking dinner.

Replace half an hour of TV watching each day with a half an hour of listening to music. Write a song or lyrics to a song. Play music when you feel worried or anxious, start listening to music as a way to distract you. If you play an instrument, sit down and play along to a favorite artist or song. Create a favorite play list you can listen to while driving to the infertility clinic. Keep sheet music nearby that you can play or sing along to. Get a karaoke machine.

If you've had formal music lessons, take out your instrument and play for your own enjoyment. Or purchase a set of drums, a piano, an organ, a flute, keyboard, or a guitar and just bang away. Let yourself enjoy creating sound for nothing more than the joy of creating sound.

Take some time to find the music that makes you feel like nothing can stop you. Play music that makes you feel like you are on a winning momentum. Research various forms of classical music to see what best suits you. If there is a certain instrument that you love, make sure to get music highlighting that instrument's sound.

Join a drumming group, take piano or clarinet lessons, sign up for a music course at a local college. Get a CD with the sounds of the ocean, wind or other forms of nature. Listen to musical theatre if it puts you in a great mood or study the works of a favorite band, singer of composer.

673. Watch What You Watch: If the evening news brings you down, stop watching it for now. Horrible images, frightening scenes, upsetting events, are not going to help your body heal and become strong. If you get news updates on your phone, stop them if they shake you up and leave you depressed.

There is some evidence that when you are sad, your adrenals become weakened, which impacts the entire hormone system in your body.

From now on, watch movies and TV shows that make you laugh and generally leave you with an optimistic, positive, upbeat feeling.

When you feel happy, you have a better chance of keeping your adrenals strong. Organs, such as the thyroid can also be weakened by a sad mood. If not keeping up with the news makes you feel guilty, realize that you are just doing it during this time in your life. It is important to give your body a chance to feel safe and watching unsettling events that attack your feelings of safety is not what your body needs right now.

674. Begin a Mild Exercise Routine: Find an gentle exercise that gets your body movingl. Nothing too demanding or harsh. Walk three or four times a week for a half hour. Note here: once you do an IVF cycle, I would suggest stopping all extreme swimming, running and aerobic work-outs. This is not the time to push your body too hard with aerobic, running, or cardio-work-outs. Extreme exercise at this time will not aid your body in conceiving, but could negatively impact the outcome of your infertility treatments.

675. Reduce the Time You Spend Looking at Screens: Too much time on your phone, computer, television, video games affects melatonin production and throws off the circadian rhythms that lead to deep, restorative sleep. As much as you can, reduce the time you spend with the technology in your life. Don't text as much, watch as many movies or TV, or play as many video games. Try to cut your screen time down in half.

676. Move the Stress out of your Body: Take walks, dance in your living room, get a massage from a trauma release specialist.

677. Thank God Every Day for Everything Good in Your Life: Say thank you for all the beauty around you. Say many 'thank you' prayers each day. Say thank you for things you never noticed before.

678. Start Keeping A Gratitude Journal: Keeping a gratitude journal will help get in the habit of focusing on the positives in your life. Studies have shown that those who keep gratitude journals and practice gratitude experience lower blood pressure, strengthened immune systems and higher levels of positive emotions in their life.Write at least three things you are grateful for at the end of each day. Keep an eye for the subtle things that you might overlook. Don't worry about what you write—there is no right or wrong way to do this, and no one is grading you on the quality of your entries.

679. Appreciate the Special Moments in Your Life: Get a poster board and write: Moments In My Life I Appreciate. Tape it to the refrigerator. Then every day, write what you experienced that day you appreciate. It could be something as simple as 'I had a nice day at work' or 'I really enjoyed going out for pizza with my friend' or 'loved talking with Mom on the phone today.' Start keeping track of all the positive things that happened in your day—even small things you previously overlooked.

680. Get an Aquarium: Some studies have shown that looking at an aquarium reduces stress and lowers blood pressure. Major retailers often have affordable tanks that come with all the basic items you need to set up. Add a few plants in your fish tank to create a pleasing environment.

681. Sing More!: Start singing as much as you can everyday. Research has shown that singing can put you in positive state of mind and reduces depression and anxiety. The use of song as a calming influence in everyday life has taken place in cultures around the world since ancient times.

Hormones such as oxytocin and endorphins are released when we sing, and those who sing have lower levels of the stress hormone cortisol in their body. Singing also lowers blood pressure and heart rate, because when we sing oxygen enters our body. Singing has been known to increase energy levels and boost the immune system. Some believe that blocked energy in the body is released through the tonal vibrations that come from singing. When we sing, we breath differently than when we are talking.

Join a local choir or start your own singing group. Set up a karaoke machine or a microphone in an easy-to-access place in your home. Get a Wii sing-along game. Join a local chorus, show choir, or vocal group. Take singing lessons. Start a singing club with your family or friends. Choose a morning song to start your day, sing on the way to work, sing on the way to your fertility treatments—don't judge yourself or your voice, just sing!

682. Keep A Journal: Give yourself ten minutes a day to write out whatever is bothering you. For just ten minutes, let whatever is within pour out on to the paper—and then leave it there, out of your body.

683. Get A Pet: Get a dog or a cat. More and more research is showing the stress-relieving benefits of having a pet. Petting your cat, walking your dog, listening to your cat purr, caring for another living being, provides social support, stress relief, a strengthened immune system, and many other health benefits. Pets ease pain and lower blood pressure. Note: if you have a cat, once you are pregnant, you want to be sure someone else is cleaning the litter box so that you do not contract toxoplasmosis, a parasitic infection carried by cats, that can cause problems to the growing fetus. Make sure the litter box is changed daily and whoever is cleaning the litter box should wear disposable gloves.

684. Read Uplifting Books: Read books that inspire, books that relax, and books that make you smile. Read classics you enjoyed in high school. Read personal growth books that encourage positive thinking and emotional healing. Read stories that give you courage, strength and hope.

685. Pray: For me, nothing helped release my stress like prayer. Being able to pray to God is and was a grand privilege that helped me like nothing else. Being able to communicate with God was what helped me most during my journey through infertility. I prayed on the way to the clinic. I prayed while I was at the clinic. I prayed on my drive home from the clinic. I prayed while my husband gave me shots, and I prayed when I waited for news from the clinic. I prayed day and night. I prayed when I felt despair, I prayed when I felt hopeless, and prayer is what gave me the strength to continue on during the hardest, most dismal times. I thank God that He gave us the privilege of prayer.

686. Do Something You Always Wanted To Do: Sometimes stress builds up when we are forced to do things we don't enjoy or really want to do. Start doing something you really want to do – something that gets you excited and thrilled.

687. Get Creative: Set up an art expression center in your home. Keep all your art supplies in an accessible bin, container or basket. Creating art is a positive way to express your emotions and release deeply buried unconscious feelings. Paint, draw, sketch, color, sculpt, glue, sew, design. Do art projects that relieve your stress and put you into a state of flow. Don't critique your work, but use these mediums as a way to release and express. If you get the urge to put your fingers in paint, smoosh away. Draw the tree outside your window. Cartoon, knit a blanket, make a collage.

Buy some coloring books and color. Make I-Love-You posters for your friends and family. Buy a journal and draw pictures. Make a colorful mosaic. Stencil, quilt, use stickers. Make greeting cards, draw animals, do collages, take your photographs and create collages of pictures and words.

688. Take a Vacation: Consider taking a vacation, a mini-vacation, or a one or two night getaway to a nearby area. If you are doing an IVF or IUI, it might help to spend a week before or after at a local beach, lake, or beautiful inn. Only consider a vacation if it will relax, not stress you. For some people, a change of scenery and escaping everyday life can help them relax. Escaping to somewhere with natural beauty, such as an ocean, mountain or river, can be very soothing.

689. Do Something Nice for Someone: Helping another person is a great way to relieve stress. When we do altruistic deeds, we experience a 'helper's high' which lowers our stress levels and improves our health. Doing kind deeds triggers our brain's reward circuity—and 'feel-good' chemicals like dopamine and endorphin are released. Buy a friend flowers, make cookies for an elderly neighbor, treat your mother to lunch, knit a blanket for a local homeless shelter, write a loving letter or card. Set a goal that you will do one kind deed a week – or everyday if possible. Kind deeds can include writing a poem for someone special, putting together a healthy fruit basket, putting a coin in an expired meter, paying the toll for the person behind you, dropping a favorite coffee off for a friend, creating a recipe book for someone who wants to learn to cook, writing a thank you note to a teacher or professor who changed your life, weeding someone's garden, cleaning someone's house, making a bagged lunch for someone. Doing something nice for someone can cost nothing to very little, but can make someone in your life feel happier, loved and thought of.

690. Smile as Much As You Can: Then smile some more.

691. Join A Group: Join a book club, knitting club, garden club or some other activity that gives you a chance to be with people.

692. Spend Time With Others: We are happier when we spend time with others. Even if you are super busy, try to make some time every day to enjoy tconversation and companionship of others. If you find yourself alone a lot, try to invite someone over at least once a week. Make a lunch date, meet in a park for a picnic, go walking or shopping together.

693. Distract Yourself: Distraction can be a way to alleviate stress. Instead of sinking into feelings of stress, start distracting yourself with fun, interesting activities. Learn cake decorating and donate cakes to brides. Start a bird sanctuary in your yard. Volunteer to beautify your town.

Learn to knit, crochet, or do needlepoint, and with each stitch, say positive words like "love" "miracle" "safety." Get a greenhouse and become an expert gardener. When I was going through infertility treatments, I kept a seed catalog by my bed that I looked at every night. Somehow, looking at all the varieties of vegetables and flowers calmed me tremendously. Try difficult puzzles. Learn an instrument. Take singing lessons. Write a book. Create a new cartoon. Photograph every tree in your town. Learn to make jewelry. Make scrapbooks for friends. Learn a new language. Go to local plays or musicals. Offer to make costumes or set designs for a local theatre company. Volunteer at a local animal shelter. Join a local singing group.

Learn a new language or about every animal native to your area. You get the idea: distract, distract, distract. Put your brain into something that will give you a break from thinking about what stresses you.

694. Write One Love Note a Day: A love note can be written to anyone in your life you care about, your sweetie, a best friend, a former co-worker you lost touch with, or a teacher you had as a child. The goal is to spread love, appreciation, and good will.

695. Massage Can Help Release Stress: Massage can help release stored memories impacting the body. So get a massage or give a massage! Either way, you'll find yourself a lot more relaxed.

696. Cuddle More: Cuddle with your spouse, your pets, your Mom and Dad, your best friend. Hug, hug, hug. Hold hands. Let yourself touch and be touched. Experience the power of a good long cuddle.

697. Don't Forget To Kiss" Yup, kissing relieves stress too!

698. Do Things That Made You Happy As A Child: Your original self holds many keys to what makes you authentically happy. This part of you knows what genuinely feeds her soul, without all the adult voices and restrictions telling her what she is suppose to do or suppose to like. Ask yourself: what did I love to do most as a child? What activities, places, games, hobbies made me totally relax and lose track of time? Try to bring some of your childhood passions into your life now.

699. **Freeing Your Body from the Traumas and Painful Memories That Might Be Destroying Your Fertility:** Our body is a walking history of our life. There is always a very strong and direct relationship between your emotional life and your physical health. You may not realize it, but trauma and painful experiences in your life can impact your fertility in a very significant way.

Your body contains and records all the traumatic and painful experiences you have endured. It then stores these traumas and sad memories in your cells and tissues.

Traumas, from rape or incest, to being bullied, criticized or rejected, can form negative pockets of energy in our cells and organs. Our bodies remember and trap feelings of fear, sadness, rejection, loneliness, betrayal, abuse, or disrespect in our cells. Our vitality and overall health is severely weakened once these negative pockets of energy inhabit our body. Even if a trauma occurred long ago, its negative energy can remain stuck in our cells for decades.

Our brain produces neuropeptides in response to our emotions, and these peptides interact with the cells in our body, firmly connecting our mind, emotions and body. The feelings and thoughts then trigger physiological responses in our body that affect the chemical and neurological balance of the hormones involved in reproduction.

Never underestimate the brutal and destructive power that traumatic and upsetting life experiences can have on your fertility. Since everything we have experienced since birth accumulates within us, to regain our health and fertility, we need to release and let go of these trauma pockets in our body that weaken us.

By releasing trauma pockets in the body, we are giving our body a chance to be restored to its true fertility potential.

When you release trauma, you are giving your body a chance to let go of the negative energy pockets stuck in the body.

Once these negative energy pockets are released, our bodies are free and unburdened from energy-draining emotions like hurt, anger, grief or shock.

Letting go, moving forward, forgiving ourselves and others, are all part of the release that is needed so that the traumas stuck in our body can no longer impact our infertility in a negative way.

Do not ignore this aspect of healing. You might have gone through a trauma or an extreme emotion that is altering the state of your body and ultimately stealing your fertility.

Here are some ways to rid your body of the traumas, painful memories and destructive emotions that could be interfering with your body reaching its maximum health potential and your right to have a baby:

700. One of the best and most powerful ways to release and unblock emotional traumas that have physically lodged themselves within your cells and tissues is through body work. Various forms of holistic treatments are available that can unblock emotional traumas. These include: chiropractic adjustments, myofascial release, cranio sacral therapy, Somato Emotional Release, deep tissue massage, trauma release massage, neuromuscular therapy, Neuro Emotional Technique, Thought Field Therapy. Zero Balancing, therapeutic touch, reflexology, kinesiology, fascia release, trauma touch therapy, Somatic Experiencing, EFT, therapeutic body work, emotional release bodywork, or light therapy. You can do an online search using these terms, adding your city or town, to see what is available in your area.

701. Consider applied kinesiology, a very powerful form of trauma release. It can be done by a kinesiologist, chiropractor or other holistic practitioner skilled in kinesiology, also known as applied kinesiology.

First, write a list of the traumatic and painful events you have experienced in your life, including names of the people who have hurt you. Give this list to a kinesiologist and ask that they muscle test each item on your list. If the kinesiologist finds that you are storing trauma associated with a certain person or experience, they can then apply an activator instrument that looks like a small, hand-held gun type mechanism, to release the emotion or trauma at its location in your body. This is a non-invasive treatment that can help you let go of long-held traumas and painful memories. If you have gone through a lot in your life, you may want to consider doing at least three or four treatments, or going on a weekly basis.

702. Homeopathy and flower essences can be used also as a way to release traumas within the body.

703. Write the experiences and events in your life that caused you a great deal of grief, trauma and fear, put them in an envelope, seal them and say goodbye to them. Mail them to an unknown address or to yourself. In these letters, say what you need to say and stand up for your right to voice out loud whatever you feel needs to be said. Your memories do not have to stay locked up inside of you. You have a right to write letters stating the truth of your pain. Even if you blame yourself or think whatever happened is your fault, trust me, whatever happened is not your fault—and feelings of shame need to be sent on their way—because you have a right to your emotions, a right to your anger, and shame no right to keep you prisoner any longer.

704. Write down all your painful memories, burn them in a fire and bury the ashes. You can do this outdoors in a fire pit, a bonfire, or in an indoor fireplace. You can do this alone, or with family and friends. Whatever you choose, it is a chance for you to physically see the end of the painful memories in your life. As they burn, consider these memories as disappearing so now you can allow vibrant fertility in your life. Throw the ashes of these memories into the ocean or bury them. The hold these traumas have over you is now gone.

705. Write a letter to yourself that gives you permission to say goodbye to your painful memories. When writing this letter, show love, compassion, forgiveness, and kindness to yourself. Let yourself know it is safe and okay to let go of the traumas of the past—that you are not safe by holding on and reliving these traumas over and over again. Let yourself know that you are not to blame for these events, nor should you keep holding yourself hostage to their power because of misguided shame you might be carrying.

706. Pray about these old memories and ask God that their hold on you be released so that your body can heal and move forward.

707. When you swim, walk or work-out, imagine that you are releasing and sweating away toxic, negative patterns in your body. For example, if you are taking a walk, with each step repeat: I am walking away from my pain, I am walking away from my pain, I am walking away from my pain. If you swim, with each lap affirm: My traumas are floating away. My traumas are floating away. My traumas are floating away.
Or you could say: My hurt is being washed away, my hurt is being washed away, my hurt is being washed away. Exercise can be a way to physically release emotional pain.

708. Write letters to the people in your past who hurt you or let you down. You never have to mail them, but in writing to them, you will energetically be releasing some of your pent-up feelings. Pour out your emotions, especially if there are people or incidents you think of often. Don't do this exercise if you have already moved past painful incidents in your life, because regurgitating old memories sometimes resurrects the pain and makes it worse. But if you find anger, sadness or other emotions pertaining to these incidents coming up often, then it is time for some cleansing and releasing. Don't be embarrassed that you are still hurt by an incident that occurred decades ago, or one that may not seem significant to others. If it hurt you and you still think or dream about it, then it deserves to be acknowledged and released.

We humans feel deeply, and we should not be ashamed of our sensitivity, our emotions or the impact that negative, toxic people and events can have on our lives.

709. Volunteer to help others who have suffered or been violated in the same way you were. Helping others is a very powerful way to heal yourself. For example, if you are a victim of some form of childhood abuse, find a way to help other victims of abuse. Or if you need to heal from bullying, volunteer to help stop bullying in your area. Empowering and helping others is a form of taking back your own power. By using your energy and insight to heal others, you will also begin to heal yourself.

710. Write a play starring yourself as a main character and tell the story of how this character releases her sad memories and goes on to give birth to a beautiful baby. You may want to act out this play before very trusted family and friends, or it might be a play for you alone to enjoy. Either way is fine. Just remember: don't be afraid to write a happy ending to this story.

711. Buy a bouquet of balloons, write your painful memories, tape them to the balloons, and then let them go one-by-one, saying goodbye to the negative impact these events had on your life.

712. Plant a garden and name each flower a positive emotion growing within your body, such as joy, self-love, self-acceptance, an ability to see beauty, or an ability to experience joy. As your flowers grow, see them as a physical manifestation of the positive emotions growing within you.

713. Write a song about the memories that weigh you down, but be sure to end the song with your letting go and moving past these memories, and on to the life you desire, surrounded by your children.

714. Write to characters in literature or history and tell them your life story. Select characters that you feel may have experienced some of the same difficult experiences you have. Ask for their advice and support in moving on to the next stage of your life. Then, write back to yourself as these characters, giving you support and advice.

715. Take a dance class and utilize the motion of dance to release toxic emotions.

716. Paint a picture of the emotional pain that lives inside your body. Name the pain. As you paint, let your inner knowing come forward to paint where your cells have stored these traumas. Use colors that express your pain. Paint pictures of the energy trapped in your cells being healed. Paint positive images of peace and joy entering your cells and tissues, allowing your fertility to blossom within you.

717. Aim to forgive. Aim to forget. Aim to accept all the imperfections in this world and still see the beauty around you. Aim to forgive even those who don't deserve your forgiveness. You might start a forgiveness journal, and each day write: I forgive _____, I forgive _____. Allow yourself to feel the relief and joy that forgiving another—even someone totally undeserving—can bring. It is understandably hard, but you deserve a future free of the pain and anger that not forgiving will bear upon you.

718. Buy or make yourself a blanket of safety. Make a blanket that symbolizes being safe—using colors, pictures, images, quotes and fabrics that give you a feeling of safety. You could make a blanket with pictures of people and places that soothe you and make you feel loved. Use material that you find pleasing and welcoming to touch. Or buy a blanket that appeals to you—it can be a kid's blanket, a lovely floral blanket, a big cozy blanket—and call it your 'safety' blanket. Sew some words on the blanket, such as 'It Is Safe For Me To Have A Baby' or 'I am Safe.' During times of stress or sadness, wrap yourself in this blanket and let yourself feel safe. Envision this blanket providing you safety from the pains of the past.

719. It is time to give yourself the empathy you deserve, whether you ever received it from others or not. If you find yourself thinking: I am insignificant, I am a failure, I am unlovable, I can't trust anyone, I am broken, I don't deserve to be happy, you need to replace these statements with: I am significant. I am a success. I am lovable. I can trust good people. I am strong and whole. I deserve to be happy.

720. Spend some time looking for what positives may have come from the traumas in your life. Are you a kinder person because of the cruelties you experienced? Are you more sensitive to the feelings of others because your feelings were disgarded? Are you a good listener because you know what it is like not to be listened to? Do you try not to hurt the feelings of others because of the betrayals and rejections you experienced? Do you look for the good in others because the constant criticism you received was so painful? Did your negative life experiences make you more determined? Hard-working? Self-sufficient? Intuitive? Wise? Forgiving? Empathetic? Generous? Write down all the ways you are a nicer, kinder, stronger, person because of difficulties you endured. Let yourself see the positives that these traumas brought you—not because you deserved to have these traumas happen, but because your body deserves to start feeling some peace.

721. Next time a traumatic memory comes into your mind, give yourself support by repeating words like: 'I am safe' or 'life is beautiful.' Other supportive statements you can repeat include: Love Is Here. Love Is Now. Love Is With Me.

722. Your story deserves to be told. Write it, videotape it, share it with others, blog it, say it. Tell it in the form of a book, a play, a journal, an essay, a musical or in song. Let yourself be heard. Share it with friends, family or strangers. As you tell your story, make sure that you note the gifts, values and strengths you maintained despite the hurt you endured.

723. Write a Declaration of Independence from your pain...stating your inalienable right to happiness, peace, feelings of security, safety and fertility! Then sign the document and make it official: you are free. You might even want to have a signing ceremony, with a fancy document and pen, making your freedom from emotional pain official!

724. Get in touch with the beliefs that sprung up within you due to the pain you experienced that might be in some way holding you back. Begin seeing those beliefs as counterfeit balloons that need to be popped! Actually, go out and get some balloons, write these limiting and constricting beliefs on the balloon and then pop them!

725. Begin to live a lifestyle where your vitality and adaptive energy can be restored, so that you have the energy to release the traumas in your body. Make sure to eat and juice a lot of greens to better alkalize your body, which can help give you the energy you will most need to heal from life's injustices and traumas.

726. Ground your energy by getting in close contact with the earth. Walk barefoot outside. Put your hands in water. Start gardening. Your body needs the healing the earth itself can provide.

727. Flood your life with positive experiences, positive words, positive images, and positive events. It has been said that the mind can only hold one thought at once. That being said, try pouring more joy into your life than you ever have before. Plan a party for someone you love, or a child at a group home, or a loved one nearing a big milestone. Learn a new skill that puts you into a state of flow. Plan a wonderful trip to a location you have always wanted to visit. Repeat the words: Life is beautiful. Life is beautiful. Life is beautiful...about 100 times a day.
Buy a bouquet of flowers for someone every week. Plant 1,000 tulips in your backyard. Start a band. Write a musical. Bake a different flavor cupcake every week and give them to strangers.

You get the idea. Fill your life with so many positive, generous acts and experiences that you tip the scales towards joy more than you ever have before.

728. Let yourself feel and then take action. Acknowledge your feelings. Then commit to an action that will make a difference in your life and in the lives of others who may be suffering too. No act is too small if you can relieve the pain of another who is suffering.

729. Write a congratulations card to yourself. Congratulate yourself on how you endured so much and how you are not allowing traumas from the past to hold you down anymore.

730. Discovering The Hidden Beliefs That Might be Holding You Back from Getting Pregnant: You may find this hard to believe, but hidden within your subconscious could be some negative perceptions of pregnancy, childbirth and motherhood that are holding you back from having a baby, without you even knowing it.

You may have some hidden fears or beliefs about becoming a mother that conflict with your desire to have a baby.

Sometimes, the body can hold two very different desires at once. One part of us wants one thing, another part of us wants another.

Consciously, you may want to become a mother more than anything in the world. Subconsciously, you may have fears that are making it hard for your conscious wishes to come true. These two very different parts of you could be playing a tug of war: who will win? Who will get their way? Whose needs will be met? This conflict can make it hard for us to really commit and do the work needed to get what we want.

This tug of war steals energy away from what your body really needs to be doing—and that is healing and getting pregnant.

Ultimately, the goal should be that all the different parts of you are working harmoniously together and have the same goal: to conceive a baby.

Deep fears and childhood issues sometimes need to be acknowledged, listened to and healed so you can move forward in having a child. It is important that you discover and acknowledge all your feelings and beliefs about becoming a mother—even the ones that are not all warm and fuzzy. Our conscious self might want something, but if our subconscious does not want it, it could be off doing a dance of its own.

If your subconscious doesn't want something, your body could follow suit.

Subconscious fears about pregnancy, child birth or raising a child could even at times influence your hormones and the physical processes required for conception.

Does having doubt, fear, or hesitance about having children mean you won't be a great mother? Not at all. Millions of great Moms once had doubts or fears about becoming a mother. Millions more worried about pregnancy, childbirth and how their life would change. Embarking on a new life path naturally brings up feelings of doubt and fear.

To find out what your subconscious really thinks about getting having a child, start by asking yourself what you think about becoming a mother, and then write down whatever response comes from you without editing yourself. Allow your subconscious to voice its feelings on the subject without judgment or criticism.

Negative feelings or beliefs left unexpressed or unresolved hold considerable energy which can block conception. If you ignore your subconscious, it might stage a rebellion within your body—not allowing you to get pregnant because it wasn't given the respect and attention it deserved.

Begin by writing: "I will become pregnant soon" or "My womb is ready to receive" and then after you write that, start writing whatever comes up from deep within. Let whatever comes up from within you come up, come out and be heard. Write without editing or judging what you are writing. Do not consciously think about what is coming up, or try to force something you don't really feel or think. Just write.

This exercise can help you uncover what you are feeling about your infertility on many levels. It can also reveal if there is a part of you that wants to sabotage your efforts to become pregnant, or feels that you are not worthy of a baby. By knowing your innermost feelings, you can then work on bringing together the different emotions within you, so that you can achieve your goal. Later on, reread what you wrote and thank your subconscious for opening up.

Try not to judge your subconscious, even if what comes up is not exactly what you want to hear.

You could also write down the words: 'I deserve to have a baby' and then type or handwrite whatever comes up. Remember: No judging. No editing. No thinking this out. Write without restraint and let your deep internal self say what it needs to say.

Other writing prompts include:

• My body is ready to conceive and give birth to a baby
• It is safe to have a baby
• I deserve to have a baby
• I am good enough to be a mother and give birth to a baby
• My body is capable of giving birth
• A woman like me deserves to be a mother
• I am ready to be a mother and have children
• It is safe for me to become a mother
• Being a mother is a good thing for me

Honestly listening to every part of yourself shows your courage, because you are not going into denial.

Every part of you needs deserves to be listened to so they can all work together. If you ignore the needs of your subconscious, it could sabotage all the hard work you are doing to get pregnant.

Here are some questions to ask yourself, write responses to, and spend some time thinking about.

731. Are you afraid of repeating the same mistakes your parents made?: Do you fear repeating some of the negative and dysfunctional family patterns you grew up with? Do you sometimes find yourself thinking, 'when I become a parent, I never want to do to my child what my parents did to me' or 'I never want to put my kids through what my parents put me through.'

732. Are you scared of becoming a mother?: Do you have fears about becoming a mother, such as or 'I'm afraid of who I will become when I have a child' or 'I'm afraid I don't have what it takes to be a good Mom' or 'I'm afraid I won't be able to care for my child properly.'

733. Are you worried about losing some of your me-time once you have a baby?: Are there aspects of your life that you really like that you are worried you will lose once you have a baby?

734. Do you fear that once you become a mother, you will turn into your own mother?: Did your Mom behave or act in a way that you don't want to repeat and hurt you a lot as a child? Or did your Mom do things that you promised yourself you would never do? Did you long ago make a silent pact with yourself that you would never become your mother?

735. Do you sometimes feel infertility is a deserved punishment, either from yourself or from God, for something you've done or didn't do, in the past?: Could infertility be something you think you deserve to suffer? Did you do something, or not do something, you believe merits you being infertile?

736. Do you feel God is mad at you?: Do you feel God is judging you harshly for something you did in your past that you still feel guilty about?

737. Were you a victim of physical, sexual abuse or emotional abuse? Did you have an abusive parent?: Do you ever fear that you will become an abusive parent like they were? If so, you might fear repeating negative family patterns.

738. Did you ever experience a trauma that has left you feeling unsafe and weary of new experiences?: Are you open to new experiences or does doing something for the first time unnerve you? Do you often feel scared and worried about your safety?

739. Are you a bit of a control freak?: Do you need to control everything in your life? Or are you able to let life flow naturally towards you? Does the idea of having a baby make you feel too out of control?

740. Do you feel you really deserve a baby?: Or do you feel unworthy of this joy? Is there something about who you are, or what you have done or experienced in life, that makes you think someone like you doesn't deserve a baby? Do you feel worthy of getting what you want?

741. Does yearning for something feel more natural and comfortable than actually getting what you want?: Have you spent a lot of your life yearning? Are you the type of person who feels more comfortable when you are yearning, wanting or suffering over something you can't have?

742. Are you more comfortable when you are the one giving, rather than the one receiving?: Do things like getting a gift or a compliment make you feel uncomfortable? Are you in the habit of being able to be on the receiving end of things?

743. Do you feel confident in your body's ability to give birth, or did you ever suffer an illness or injury that has shaken your belief in what your body can do?: Do you see your body as weak and incapable? Have you ever suffered from a trauma or an illness that has left you doubting your body's strength and capability? Does physical pain of any sort bring up bad memories for you?

744. When you think of being pregnant, does the word 'fat' come to your mind?: Do you consider pregnant women beautiful or unattractive? Do you fear losing your shape or physical beauty once you have a baby? Do you fear that pregnancy will ruin your body? Do you see pregnancy as an empowering event for your body or something that will steal the hot body you are proud of.

745. Does the work of caring for a baby seem overwhelming? Are you afraid of the demands that a child will make on your life?: Do you ever see mothers with their children and think 'I could never do all that work.'

746. When you hear the word 'mother' do positive or negative images come to your mind?: Do you associate the title 'mother' with positive, loving images or negative, frightening images?

Do you think of the positive words associated with mothers, such as loving, protective, warm, or do you think of the negative connotations surrounding motherhood sometimes promoted in the media, such as being controlling or demanding?

747. Do you fear going through childbirth or did your mother go through a very hard delivery with you?: Do images of a woman screaming in pain come to your mind when you think of childbirth? Did you grow up hearing horror stories about your own birth? Did your mother talk a lot about the difficulty she had giving birth to you or a sibling? Do you have any negative thoughts about childbirth, due to media images or experiences of family or friends?

748. Did your own mother enjoy having children or did she complain about how hard it was to be a mother?: Did you grow up with a mother, or a father, who found being a parent very difficult? As a child, could you sometimes sense how frustrated or overwhelmed your parents were with raising children? Did their experience taint your view of parenthood?

749. Do you fear that your body can't survive childbirth? Does being pregnant or giving birth seem dangerous to you in any way?: On some level, do you fear you might die during childbirth? Do you think being pregnant hurts? Do you have concerns about the physical dangers of child birth? Do you see woman as being in danger when they are pregnant or give birth?

750. Do you feel ashamed because you want a baby?: Does your intense desire to be a mother make you feel ashamed? In general, do you often feel the emotion of shame, especially when it comes to your own desires and needs?

751. Do you feel capable of caring for a child and being a good mother? Did someone ever say or suggest you would be a terrible mother? Or that you are not capable of being a mother?: Sometimes people can see us in one way only, and because we've never done something, they cannot imagine us doing it.

752. Were you ever at the mercy of a female who was cruel to you?: Have you somehow equated the cruelty of a mother, stepmother or female caretaker with a role you are about to step into?

753. Have you spend a lot of your life trying not to get pregnant?: Have you told your body that it is now okay to get pregnant? Have you given your body permission to get pregnant?

754. Do you respect your feminine self and genuinely like being a woman?: Or do you see things defined as feminine as dumb, stupid or unworthy of respect? Do you respect the feminine body that has the ability to carry and give birth to a child, or is there a part of you that disrespects the feminine body?

755. Do you trust yourself enough to become a mother?: Or because of your family history or childhood experiences, do you distrust yourself?

756. Do you fear that becoming a mother will change you in a way that you don't want to change?: Do you fear having a child will change something about who you are, or a part of your personality, you value and like about yourself?

757. Do you worry a lot about having a child with birth defects?: Do you think a lot about the 'what ifs'?

758. Do you fear that you don't have what it takes to be a good mother?: Is there some aspect of your personality or character that makes you think that women like you are not cut out to be good mothers? Have friends or family ever joked that you would be a terrible mother?

759. Is your husband/partner truly the person you want to have a baby with?: Or do you have doubts about raising a child with him? Do you think your partner will be a good father or not?

760. Do you worry about certain choices you might be forced to make when you have a child, such as what religion you will raise them in, or how you will pay for college?: Do you find yourself worrying about the choices that will face you when you have a child?

761. Do you link being a mother to having to endure some type of suffering?: Did you ever, somewhere along the way, get the idea that being a mother equals some type of physical or emotional suffering?

762. Do you think having children ruined your mother's life or trapped her in some way? Do you fear becoming a Mom will trap you also?: Did you ever see your own mother as being trapped because she had children? Do you think your mother was trapped in a bad marriage because she had you? Or did she suffer economic hardship because she was raising children? Did she give up a promising career because she was a mother? Did you ever see your mother struggling and think, 'I never want to trapped like my Mom."

763. Do you fear you are too old to have a baby?: What are your views on aging? Do you sometimes think that only young women can have healthy babies?

764. Do you fear that this is an unsafe world to bring a child into?: Do you worry about bringing a child into a world with problems? Do you watch the evening news and think 'how could anyone bring a child into this world'?

765. Do you feel guilty bringing a child into this world?: Do you ever feel selfish for wanting to have a baby?

766. Do you ever feel like you can't afford a child?: Do you think a lot about how you will afford to raise children? Are you worried about the financial responsibility of raising a child?

767. Do you fear that having a child could destroy your marriage?: Do you worry that your relationship with your husband will change once you have a baby?

768. Do you worry that your sex life will end once you become a mother?: Do you think that Moms are sexy? Or do you think the sensual part of a woman disappears once she becomes a mother?

769. Do you fear that having a child will destroy your career?: Do you love working and worry a lot about how you will continue your career once you have children to take care of? Do you fear that having a child will put an end to all the other goals that are important to you?

770. Do you fear that having children will threaten some of the important relationships in your life?: Are there relationships in your life that you fear will be threatened once you have kids? Do your friends have children or are they childless?

771. Are you a perfectionist who thinks you need to be perfect and everything in your life should be perfect before you become a mother?: Do you feel you should be perfect before becoming a mother? Do you want to be a good mother so badly that a part of you believes only being perfect is good enough?

772. Do you welcome change into your life?: Or are you the type of person who fights change and finds any type of change very difficult?

773. Did your own mother abandon you, either due to divorce, death or neglect?: If you were abandoned in any way by your mother, having a child and becoming a mother yourself may bring up a lot of fear. Secretly, you may fear that you are going to be like your mother and abandon your children also. You might fear repeating your mother's negative pattern of abandonment. You might still feel so angry at the feminine role model in your life, i.e. your mother, that having anything in common with her, a.k.a. both being mothers, might be something you want desperately to avoid.

Within you, might be a little girl still longing for her mother—so much so, that becoming a mother might be something your 'little girl within' resists. Or, you might blame yourself for your mother leaving, and subconsciously you equate children with pain because on some level, you believe your mother's leaving you was justified on her part. So why would you feel comfortable having a child—when a part of you believes children deserve to be left?

774. Was one of your parents an alcoholic or drug addict?: If so, you may fear that having a child will kick off this cycle again. Maybe you blamed yourself for your parent's addiction—and now you wonder if having a child will spark an addiction within you.

775. Do you tend to shy away from responsibility?: Does the responsibility of becoming a parent scare you? Are you often scared of taking on new responsibilities in general? Do you have confidence in your ability to take on new life assignments, or do you doubt yourself?

776. Do You Say No A lot Easier And Quicker Than You Say Yes: Do you more often say no than yes?

Now that you've asked yourself these questions, here are some thoughts that might help you heal some the fears and beliefs that could be blocking your infertility:

777. You don't have to be perfect to be a good mother. Let go of the idea that for you to be a mother, it is perfect or bust. There are millions of kind, loving mothers who are not perfect in any way and make lots and lots of mistakes—and yes, their kids turned out fine. You will make mistakes and that is okay. Let go of the notion of perfect. It doesn't exist. You are not perfect right now, nor will you be once you have a child…and that is perfectly okay. Millions of children grow up to be happy, functioning adults and none of them had perfect parents. Remind yourself that being a good mother is one who tries hard, admits their mistakes and learns from them.

778. If you feel your parents made a lot of mistakes in raising you, remind yourself that learning from the mistakes of others is something we humans can do very well. If your parents behaviors or choices hurt you deeply and resulted in your having a difficult childhood, set out to make a conscious decision to make different choices than they made.

Remember: you are not your mother and father. You can learn from their good choices and from their bad ones. You are not a prisoner of your family history or family patterns. You can do it differently. You have choices about how you will live your life. You are not pre-destined to do what your parents did.

You can educate yourself through the thousands of books on healthy parenting. You can find a person you consider a good parent to mentor you. You can do a form of therapy that heals you and helps you formulate a plan of how you will handle some of the challenges your parents didn't handle so well. You can pray to God everyday to be a decent, kind and loving parent.

You have the right to write your own life script, one very different from your parents.

You've got the key—now let yourself out.

There are resources within you and in the world around you that can help you be the parent you want to be, regardless of the family you come from. You can acknowledge the weaknesses that existed within your family—and then you can work hard to avoid the behaviors and choices that fueled the negative behaviors.

Simply making the decision that you will try to be a loving, kind and hard-working parent is a great start. If you feel you face a special challenge due to your family background, such as a history of alcoholism or sexual abuse, don't be ashamed to look for help in breaking destructive family patterns.

779. Remember that being a mother does not mean you have give up all the other parts of yourself that you value. There are millions of mothers who live a life that is true to who they are. Many mothers continue being artists, writers, poets, doctors, lawyers, teachers and whatever else they choose to be, while raising their children.

You have a right to hold on to the parts of you that you hold sacred and dear, and in being true to yourself, you will be setting a great example for your child. While being a mother does require hard work and sacrifice, it should not mandate giving up all the parts of yourself that you cherish.

780. You are allowed to have more than one dream. It is okay to dream of being a mother—and okay to have other dreams too. More than one life dream is allowed.

781. If you worry about losing me-time once you have a baby, create a plan that will give you some of the alone time you need. Are there grandparents or relatives nearby who are willing to babysit? What childcare options are available to you?

Remember: you are not a bad Mom if sometimes you need time for yourself. But, you might actually enjoy spending time with your little one much more than you now realize.

782. Did your mother behave or live her life in a way that hurt you? If you fear that having a child will turn you into your mother, remember once you consciously acknowledge something and bring it into the light, its hold on you is significantly lessened. If you believe you have qualities or personality traits like your Mom that you don't want to repeat, seek help and learn how to break negative behaviors and patterns.

Be aware that no two people are exactly alike even if they are alike. Your situation and life experience doesn't have to be the same as your mothers. In fact, you can learn from your mother in what not to do. You can spend some time analyzing what your mother might have needed that would have made things easier for her. Did your mother need some type of medication to address a mental health issue?

Did she need exercise, a creative outlet outside the house, a different diet that would have better suited her needs?

You also have to realize that times have changed since you were a child, and challenges your mother faced might not even exist today.

You are not sentenced to recreate the dysfunction of your Mom if you choose not to.

783. If something within you makes you feel unworthy or undeserving of being a mother, remember that as a human being, you are worthy and this is your natural birthright.

Remind yourself daily that you deserve to have the baby of your dreams, and you don't need to be perfect to enjoy this role. Let go of the idea that you deserve punishment in any way. Love yourself, forgive yourself, and repeat: I deserve a baby, I deserve a baby, I am worthy of having a baby.

784. Many women, before becoming mothers, wonder if they are capable of caring for a baby. It is a natural concern, and yet step-by-step, day- by-day, millions of women learn how to care for their babies with great and profound knowledge, insight, strength and love. You have within you the capacity to learn and grow.

You don't need to know everything all at once. You have to trust the learning process your life as a mother will provide you with. There are hundreds of books on childcare that you can read, and you can talk and get tips from other mothers on how to care for children.

785. If doing something new feels unsafe or frightening, start saying to yourself: 'new experiences are safe for me' or 'it is safe for me to have a baby' several times a day. Often, the most frightening aspect of doing anything new is the time before you actually do it, when you are thinking about and imagining yourself doing it. Did you ever worry about something you were going to do that you never did before, but once you dived in and started doing it, a lot of the fear disappeared, because you realized it was not as hard as you thought it would be.

Many of your fears will disappear once you actually have a child. Fears of changing a diaper, feeding a baby, keeping a baby safe, will dissolve as you actually do it. Before I had children, I really believed I could not endure changing a diaper. Once I had a baby, I actually loved changing diapers and had no problem with it at all.

786. If you tend to be a control-freak or just someone who likes a measure of control in your life, set up things ahead of time that will give you a feeling of being in control. Then, trust. Just trust. It will be okay. You may need to learn how to let life happen, rather than always trying to control.

787. If you've had health issues in the past, remind yourself that the human body is strong and resilient. If there are aspects of childbirth that worry you, talk with your doctor about planning a birth experience that you will feel safe with. It is okay to do whatever is necessary to reduce the pain you will experience. No guilt please on that one.

While some women are okay with no pain medication, other women welcome relief from the pain involved with childbirth—and that is perfectly okay too. Even if your mother had a very difficult delivery with you, remind yourself that times have changed, medical procedures have advanced, and that you will probably have a different doctor and experience than she had.

788. If you worry constantly that you are not going to be a good mother, relax and take the pressure off yourself. In the media, we are presented two very different versions of motherhood. One is the perfectly sweet, kind, loving mother and the other is the evil, controlling, wicked selfish mother. The reality is most mothers are not all-goodness or all-evil. Take the pressure off yourself. Yes, you have a responsibility to treat your child with love and kindness, but nobody is perfect—even the most perfect of mothers are not perfect. A side note here: this does not give you permission to be abusive, cruel, neglectful, or dismissive to your child, but it does give you permission to be human.

789. If sometimes you fear that having a child will be too much work for you and that you are not capable, repeat and think about these affirmations: I am capable of being a Mom. I am capable of learning. I am capable of working hard when I need to. I am capable of trying again when I make a mistake. I am capable of improving on skills I already have and acquiring skills I don't have.

790. If you have worked hard to be in shape and fear that pregnancy and childbirth will ruin your body, remind yourself that there are many, many hot Moms out there. Women who work out and eat well usually look great, whether they have no kids or five kids. The habits that put you in good shape will still be available to you, whether you are a Mom or not. Think of it this way: when you are 80 years old, do you want to have a human being beside you or a picture of how great you looked way back when.

Start to see pregnancy and childbirth as an empowering event for your body, where you get to tap into your body's full potential.

791. Start thinking about all the fun you will have with your child, rather than the pain and loss you imagine you will experience. Spend time thinking about what you will gain when you have a child, rather than what you will lose. Start thinking about all the positive changes that come with having a baby, rather than dwelling on what you think will be negative changes in your life. Positive changes can include: having someone to love, having another person to become stronger for, having someone to teach, nurture and do lots of fun things with.

Spend some time thinking about all the fun, life-enhancing things you will do with your child. Focus on the pleasure, not the pain, of having babies. Think about cuddling and holding your baby, baking with your little girl, playing baseball with your son, building with blocks, reading stories, spending a day at the beach, going to a park.

Think about the traditions, hobbies, and family heritage you can share with your child. Think about the beauty of creating a family, and having as your legacy your role as a mother.

 When the fears start to invade your head, turn it around by thinking about the positives. Maybe even create a scrapbook entitled: The Fun I Will Have With My Child and cut out pictures of all the fun, wonderful things you plan to do together. Look at this book often, so anticipation and joy replaces the fear.

792. If your mother didn't enjoy being a mother, it doesn't mean you will feel the same way. Think about it: is your life right now exactly like your mothers? Are you exactly like your mother? Are your circumstances identical to your mothers? When you have children, will your life be just like hers? Probably not. Repeat: I am not my mother. I will live the life I want to live, not the life my mother lived. You can also spend time analyzing what aspects of motherhood your might have found hard, and do what you can in advance to prepare yourself for such challenges.

793. If you find yourself excessively worrying about things like will my child have a birth defect, stop, read up on all the things you can do to maximize your chances for a healthy baby. Find out what foods you can eat and supplements you can take before you get pregnant, such as folic acid. Schedule 'worry time' once a week, rather than allowing worry to crowd your thoughts on a daily basis.

794. If you have concerns about your husband being a good father, take steps to address the issue. Talk with your husband about your concerns, attend parenting classes together, read parenting books and seek male role models that can mentor your husband in his new role as a father.

795. If you worry a lot about everything, just stop. That's it. Stop projecting into the future. You can plan. You can take positive steps to address certain concerns, but worrying about every little thing won't serve you or your child. Stop projecting into the future. Stop playing out negative scenarios. Stop focusing on all the bad stuff. Just stop.

796. When you feel overwhelmed by negative thoughts or fears, do affirmations, such as: it is safe for me to have a baby. It is safe and okay to be pregnant. Childbirth is easy for me. Childbirth is safe for me. I am looking forward to a beautiful birth experience. My baby and I will enjoy a beautiful birth experience.

797. Begin to link the idea of pleasure to being pregnant and having a baby. We as humans run towards pleasure and run away from pain. To help your subconscious get over its fears, you need to begin to convince it that having a baby will mean more pleasure in your life than pain. Do a collage with positive words and images about childbirth and motherhood. Talk to your subconscious often about all the joy, happiness and contentment you will experience as a mother. Make a list of all the activities you can look forward to doing as a mother and read this list often.

798. If you have a lot of concerns about how your life will change once you have a baby, begin a preparation plan that addresses your concerns. Bring in the support you will need. You'll feel better, more in control, and you'll see the possibilities for creating a life with your child that pays respect to your needs.

799. If you have gone through a trauma in the past that has left you feeling perpetually unsafe, begin to do body work to release the trauma so that your body can relax and let down its guard, and allow you to have a baby.

800. If your mother abandoned or rejected you in any way, you have seen the dark side of motherhood. For you to become what you may hold great anger and hatred towards, you need to try to forgive your mother, and at the same time, hold the confidence that you are going to tap into the positive side of motherhood, something perhaps your own mother never did. Rather than looking at the woman who left or rejected you as a mother, you need to see her actions as a result of who she was as a person, disconnecting the link to motherhood in any way. She did not leave you because she was a mother—she left you because she was a person with flaws, deficiencies and most likely great emotional and mental pain.

It was not motherhood or being a mother that made your mother hurt you, it was something within her that most likely manifested itself in various aspects of her life, including parts of her life that had nothing to do with being a mother.

801. Feeling afraid of a big life changer like having a baby is normal. Having some fears, wondering if you are really ready to be a mother, does not mean you are not ready—it means you are human and millions of women throughout history have gone through similar feelings of doubt, fear and hesitation, before becoming the amazing, wonderful mothers they turn out to be. Having some natural fears and apprehension is not a sign that you are not ready, capable and able to be a great mother. Believe it or not, it is completely normal and okay to desperately want a child and, be afraid and hesitant at the same time.

Feeling two conflicting emotions at once doesn't mean you are not ready to welcome and care for your baby. It just means you are human, and sometimes we are afraid of new experiences and changes in our lives.

Creative Exercises

802. Creativity is a powerful anecdote to feelings of hopelessness and depression. Doing creative activities can help you unlock and release negative energy patterns and paths in the body. Tapping into your creativity can help you transcend emotional blockages that may exist within your body.

Exploring your creativity can relax you, de-stress you, and give your body a dose of happy, healthy chemicals that can assist in healing infertility.

Here are some creative exercises and activities to try while undergoing infertility treatments:

803. Make a collage representing birth, babies, and the body's ability to conceive and have a baby.

You'll need a poster board, construction paper, or whatever kind of paper feels right to you. Cut out pictures from magazines, books, newspapers, or download and print pictures from the Internet of babies, pregnant women, along with images and words that represent what getting pregnant and having a baby means to you. Then, glue them in whatever pattern you choose on the paper or poster board of your choice.

When I was trying to get pregnant with my second child, I made a huge collage that affirmed my body's ability to get pregnant. I cut out pictures of babies and words like "the princess has arrived" and "mother love." I used lots of positive words that meant a lot to me and I personally connected to having children. My collage had pictures that represented new life emerging and the upcoming and most definite arrival of my child. I hung it in my office so I could look at it and feed off its positive energy every day. Making this collage was a very joyful experience for me, because I had been trying for over a year to get pregnant and was not successful. I was extremely depressed, but while making the collage, I entered a very optimistic and hopeful state of mind.

Every time I looked at my collage, I felt renewed hope and a surge of power—something that I needed desperately to gain back at that time. A few months later, I did become pregnant and gave birth to my beautiful son.

So, collage away. I used a huge poster board which I felt made my collage something powerful to look at. Make sure to use whatever images, pictures, words strike a personal note for you.

804. Make a collage celebrating babies. Cut out photos of babies from magazines and write something at the top like: Welcoming All Babies— Including Mine! Or: Welcome To All The Babies and My Baby Too! Put a picture of yourself in the middle of this collage along with something that represents your baby's arrival. In doing this, you'll be setting out the welcome mat for your baby's arrival and reminding yourself that babies are born everyday and soon yours will be too!

805. Make a collage on the topic of fertility. Use words and pictures that represent your body enjoying a healthy state of fertility. If you see pictures that symbolizes fertility to you, add it to your collage. Make sure to put a picture of yourself in the middle of the collage, with words like: "My Body is Fertile" or "The World Around Me Is Fertile and I Am Fertile Too" or "I Am Part of A Fertile World." Surround your picture with powerful and meaningful images of fertility that you can personally relate to.

806. Create a scrapbook titled "My Successful Journey To Motherhood" and include in it whatever pictures, quotes, experiences or items reflect your story of having children.

807. Go to a crafts store and purchase pink and blue buckets and make flower arrangements that you will have in your hospital room when you have a baby. Get flowers and decorations that you want in your room when you have a baby.

808. Play inspiring music, like the theme to the movie 'Rocky', and march around your living room, picturing your ovaries turning out a healthy baby. Play music that puts you in a state of positive expectation and joy. Allow the music to help you transcend all doubt, if even for just a few minutes. Let the music carry you into a state of being where you allow yourself to feel your dream of being a mother coming true. Play a song that represents triumph and victory as you see yourself giving birth and becoming a mother. Then, as you play this song, move, march, dance in a celebratory way that says: my baby is on the way to me soon.

809. Make a collage of all the goals and dreams in your life that came true, as a hefty reminder that good things do happen to you and will happen to you again. By reminding yourself that you can get what you want, you'll be triggering the thought of 'it happened once, it can happen again.' Along with words and images of goals and dreams that came true, include a picture of yourself next to a baby and write on the collage, "my dream of having a baby is my next dream about to come true." Hang it in a place where you can see it often.

810. Write a song about your victory over infertility. Songwriting is a way to express your feelings about having a baby in a hopeful and positive way. Write and sing a song about the triumphant way your body was able to conceive and give birth to a baby, as if it already happened. Write a song inviting your baby to find a home in your womb. Write a song to your future child about all the wonderful things you will do together. You don't have to be musically inclined to pen a song that speaks of hope and the happiness that awaits you.

811. Cut out words that describe the strength of your body and glue them onto a large piece of poster paper. Put a picture of yourself in the center of these words, which can include words like: Fertile. Reproducing. Wise. Strong. Healthy. Ripe. Hang it somewhere where you can look at it often.

012. Imagine you are a coach and let your inner fertility coach give you tips on how to get pregnant. See getting pregnant as a game and listen to what your inner coach has to say about what you need to do to win this game. You can ask your inner coach to create a playbook, with the actions needed for you to win this fertility game. Draw a picture of your inner fertility coach and write down your inner coach's five best pieces of advice. Hang it somewhere you can see it often. You know more than you think and this is a way to tap that inner knowing.

813. Make or buy a kite and write your wish to have a baby, attach it to the kite, and send the kite out into the universe. Or attach to the kite a message inviting your future child to come to you and let it go into the world. Create as many kites as you wish and send them off with whatever message about having a baby you want to send out into the world.

814. Write a story about the day your child is born. Imagine the sights, the smells, the sounds, of this beautiful experience that awaits you. Write about the faces you will see, the emotions you will experience, the feeling of touching your child for the first time. As you write, let your body feel the story as if it were a reality, that already happened.
Go into detail: what hospital will you give birth in? What words will your partner, mother, and doctor say to you on the day your child is born? What will you wear to the hospital? How will you pack your suitcase? Write as if it already happened.

815. Paint a picture of how you feel about having a baby, using colors, symbols, words and images...whatever comes up from within you about your child.

816. Draw a picture of yourself holding a baby or holding hands walking with your child. Look at the picture often as if it has already come to pass.

817. Pick a song that will be you and your child's theme song someday and play it often. Dance to it and imagine you are dancing together at your child's wedding. Imagine you are at your child's high school graduation party and you're explaining to all the guests how this was a song you played when you were wishing and hoping for the arrival of your child. Imagine dedicating this song to your child at their kindergarten or middle school graduation party. Keep a CD in your car or download on your phone and play this song often—always imagining you and your child dancing and celebrating your love for one another.

818. Write a story about your journey to have a child--and give it a happy ending. Write about how you finally got pregnant, carried full term, and delivered your baby.

819. Make a collage using images and words representing living things that reproduce, such as animals, plants, trees. Put a picture of yourself right smack in the middle of this collage, reminding yourself that you too are part of this life cycle--a living being born with the ability and right to reproduce. Write something like: All Living Creatures Reproduce And I Can Reproduce Too!

820. Write a story as told by your body about your problems getting pregnant. Have your body explain what healed it and enabled it to conceive and give birth. Don't think this out--just write whatever comes. Even if it makes no sense, let whatever your body say what it wants to say. Let your body tell the story of how you healed from infertility, whether it makes sense or not.

821. Make a collage that says 'Thank You' for all the babies that will be born on this earth in the next few years, including yours. Say thank you for the millions of births that occur every day throughout the world, including the upcoming birth of your own baby. Include pictures, images, colors and words of gratitude that express a thankful heart for the births happening everywhere at this time—and the birth that will occur in your own life soon.

822. Choreograph a dance that symbolizes your fertility. Choose a song that represents your body giving birth. Create movements that mirror this amazing journey of birth that you will soon experience. Use music, costumes and props that show your body in the state of receiving a child into your womb and then giving birth.

You could also take a dance class and ask your teacher to help you create a dance that symbolizes your journey to becoming a mother. You might want to consider taking a ballet, hip hop, jazz, belly dancing or some other type of dance class and incorporate what you learn into the dance you will create.

Once you have created your dance and chosen the music, do this dance often as an invitation for your body to follow suit. If you like, perform it for family and friends, as a way to express your fertility.

823. Make a collage showing all the ways you are a mother right now to your family, friends, and the world around you. Place a picture of yourself in the center of the collage and surround yourself with pictures and images of the way you now manifest your mothering ability. As you do this collage, let yourself see how you are ready and capable you are of being a mother, because in many ways, you have begun the mothering process.

824. Draw a rainbow with the colors you associate with birth. Put your picture in the center of the rainbow.

825. Buy a drum and beat out the news of your child's upcoming arrival. Play this drum in whatever way your body intuitively wants to play it, announcing to the world the soon-to-be arrival of your baby.

826. Take walks in natural settings as much as possible, and take pictures every time you notice the birth cycle in your environment. Say aloud, "thank you that I am part of this natural process of conceiving life and giving birth." Then, write a two-page essay on your observations regarding the birth cycle in the world around you and include your photographs in it.

827. Get a box and each day put items inside it that symbolize the gifts you are going to share with your future children. These gifts can include words that you will impart to your children, pictures of places you plan to visit together, lists of things you will do together, books you will read, hobbies you will pursue. It can also be items that symbolize spiritual and emotional gifts you plan to share with your children.

828. Make a storybook of the kind of mother you want to be. Let your inner maternal voice shine as you write, draw and paste pictures of the type of mother you plan on being to your children.

829. Write a letter welcoming your child to the world. Your letter can include your hopes and dreams for your child, favorite memories you want to share, and information about yourself. Put the letter or letters in a box with the words: Letters to My Child.

830. Buy a beautiful chest and make it your baby hope chest. Paint and decorate this chest in ways that inspire you. Then each day, put something in the chest that symbolizes your hope and confidence that your child will be born. You can put items, such as a picture of a flower that you will grow in a garden together, recipes you want to make with your child, pictures of the places you will go together, books you will to read to your children, and favorite pieces of music you want to share. Consider this box a place to put many of the dreams you have for your child and the childhood you will create for them.

831. Go somewhere in nature, such as your backyard, and put your hands in dirt and feel the pulsating life that lives right beneath you each day. Or buy a big pot and fill it with soil. Sit outside and let your hands dig in the soil and feel the rich fertility of the soil, reminding yourself that you are as fertile as this soil. As you feel the soil, say: I am as fertile as this soil.' Do this often.

832. Invite family and friends who have supported you in your journey to have a baby to participate in a parade, where you all will march through a forest or your backyard, singing songs affirming that your body is healing and able to have a baby. Invite everyone to make posters welcoming your future child.

Let your friends and family nurture, love and support you, as you state aloud your firm conviction that your body can and will conceive and give birth--and that, yes, you will find a way to fulfill your desire to parent.

833. Write a message to your future baby, put it in a bottle, and release it into the ocean. Ask whoever finds the bottle to send you positive thoughts in your quest to have a baby.

834. Plant a garden dedicated to your future child. Give your garden a name and a theme. Put figurines of children in the garden, symbolizing that you are welcoming living beings into your life. Keep a journal about your experiences with this garden. Then, take a picture of your garden and put it aside as a gift to give to your future child.

835. Get a bunch of washable paints and allow your body to completely relax as you release your feelings about giving birth through color and finger movement. The painting doesn't have to look like anything, but simply is a way to express.

836. Create a birthing rainbow with colors that heal you. At the end of the rainbow, draw a picture of your baby or cut out a picture of a baby and place it there. Look at these healing colors daily--and then look at that baby at the end of the rainbow. Visualize these colors healing your body and helping you produce your 'baby at the end of the rainbow.'

837. What do you look forward to doing with your future children? Make a scrapbook with all the fun activities you are excited to do with your kids. This can include games you want to play, brochures of places you want to visit, and arts and craft projects you want to do together.

838. Every morning, step outside your door, raise your arms to the sky and say, "I am ready for my baby!" "I welcome my baby' 'Thank you for my baby.'

839. For one day, act as if you are pregnant. Eat, drink, walk, sleep and move like you are pregnant. Talk as if you are already pregnant. Say out loud, "I am pregnant." Let your body think it is pregnant. At the end of the day, write about how you felt being pregnant.

Write it as if it was a reality. Call this essay: Today I Am Pregnant.

840. Buy a dollhouse and work on furnishing and decorating it for your future child. Make the house something either a boy or girl would enjoy, perhaps making some rooms 'superhero' themes and other rooms more of a girl-oriented theme.

841. Design the backyard of your dreams for your future child. Make a collage with pictures of swing sets, pools, doll houses and more.

842. Sing! Sing! Sing your way to pregnancy! Select songs that imbue you with the feelings of joy and hope. Have the words of the songs in front of you, and each day, sing them aloud. As you sing, envision yourself pregnant and giving birth to your baby. Choose songs that reflect your positive vision of becoming a mother.

843. Create a special dance for you and your husband. Choose a song that makes you both feel very hopeful about having a baby. Choreograph this dance as a moving, living symbol of how you two will make a baby together.

844. Paint some dishes for your future child and imagine that someday your child will eat delicious meals you prepared on them.

845. Create positive, hopeful greeting cards for other women experiencing infertility. Make sure these cards offer words of hope and healing, and donate them to an infertility clinic, or give as a gift to a friend also experiencing infertility. Or leave them in the waiting room of the clinic you go to, as a way to share and impart hope to others.

846. Get your camera and go out and take pictures that are Proof That Miracles Happen. Then, make a photo collage with the title: Proof That Miracles Happen. Make sure one of the pictures is of you wearing a t-shirt that says: I am pregnant!

847. Write a one-woman play about your experiences with infertility. But....end the play with you talking about how you became pregnant and had a baby! Speak this aloud with conviction and positive belief.

848. Begin a daily diary that you will give to your child someday. Start your entries by writing: To My Child or Dear Baby and share with your future child whatever you like to share about your day or your life.

849. Set up a place in your home where you can paint your body healing from infertility. Paint whatever colors, forms, images come to you. Let your inner artist paint whatever it wants to express about the physical and emotional healing your body needs to experience to become pregnant. If it helps, paint the pain, emotional wounds and physical parts of your body that are calling out for healing in your infertility journey.

850. Knit, crotchet or sew blankets, hats and clothes for your baby. Allow yourself to picture your baby wearing them as you create them. Or, begin to sew maternity clothes for yourself, including what you want to wear the day you give birth. Sew clothes that include patches with sayings like: 'can't wait to meet you!' 'Mommy loves you!' 'So excited to see you!' on them.

851. Make a quilt representing your journey through infertility with your desired destination of becoming a mother as part of your journey. Create a quilt that is positive and hopeful, and conveys the idea and energy that yes—you will become pregnant and have a baby soon! Don't worry if your quilt is not perfect. Be sure to choose images that align with a positive vision of your baby's arrival. You could also make a wreath, with items such as rattles, bath toys, pacifiers, teething rings, representing your baby's arrival. (p.s.: when your baby arrives, hang this beautiful wreath on your hospital door!)

852. Create artwork for your future children's bedroom. Draw or paint pictures. Put together a book of pictures with quotes you want to share with your child.

853. **Making Your Home Into A Fertility Nesting Center:**
Transporting yourself to an island paradise tomorrow may not be possible, but creating a world at home that is a nurturing incubator for you and your baby is possible. Your home can be a helper in your fertility. It can be a nest where you feel safe enough to conceive, receive, give birth and care for your babies.

Sometimes, just a simple change can turn a home into a loving nest: painting a room a color you love, putting a sweet teddy bear or cozy quilt on your bed, hanging a photograph that calms or inspires you. Envision yourself as a mother bird preparing a nest for her eggs she must keep safe and warm. Feeling safe and in a nest will help you at this time, since the body finds it easier to procreate when it does not feel threatened or in a state of fight or flight. Look around your house and ask yourself: Do I like it here? Do I feel safe here? Do I feel like I can safely keep and 'hatch my eggs here'? Try to find ways to make your living space one in which you feel safe and comfortable. This could include: displaying a tea cup or doll collection, hanging photographs of people, places and memories that leave you feeling happy and warm inside.

Create a room that reminds you of things you loved as a child. How about a shelf in your kitchen with Raggedy Ann and Andy dolls? Or a 'Disney Dreams Come True' room with memorabilia from the various Disney princesses if that is something you love.

Walk around your home and try to find ways to increase the feelings of safety, joy and comfort. Even if you don't live in an ideal setting or particularly like where you live, there are small things you can do to make your home feel more like a warm incubator for yourself and your baby. Start by looking around home, and ask yourself: where do my eyes spend most of their time? Notice where your eyes go each day—during breakfast, dinner, where you watch TV, and try to make your where your eyes spend their time more conducive to positive feelings. Whatever areas of your home get your 'eye' time offer key opportunities for healing.

For example, if you often find yourself sitting in a certain room, looking at a certain wall, could you hang a positive saying or beautiful picture that inspires you or just make you feel happy? Example: When I was trying to get pregnant, I hung a picture of a little girl playing with a bunny in my bedroom. The picture made me feel soft and hopeful, even during very painful moments. Ask yourself: what could I bring into my home that would bring pleasure to my eyes, ears and body each day? Think about items you could put in your home that would bring you a renewed sense of joy every time you look at them.

In whatever ways you can, make your home a place of healing, a nest where you can rest and rejuvenate as you prepare to conceive, an environment where you can access the positive emotions within you.

Here are some ways to turn your home into a comforting nest for you and your baby:

854. Color: What colors make you sparkle? What colors give you a feeling of peace? Don't worry about what colors are popular or 'in' right now—think about how different colors make you feel.

Then, put colors in your home that give you the type of feelings you are looking for. If certain colors lift your spirits, bring those colors into your life. Look around: could you paint your bathroom a brilliant orange, the kitchen a soft pink, your living room a relaxing lavender. Think out of the box. Are you in the mood for bright, vibrant colors, like green or orange that bring about a friendly, happy feeling? Some color experts believe the color orange can help balance the adrenal glands, red provides energy and vitality to the ovaries, and violet is nurturing to the pituitary glands. Pay close attention to what colors you are drawn to and then bathe your home in these beautiful colors.

855. Photographs: Photographs are a powerful way to relive positive, happy memories. Instead of keeping your pictures locked away in boxes, or on your phone, print them out, buy a few frames and hang them throughout the house. Take photographs of places in nature that soothe you and people that you love. Display photographs that are reminders of life's beautiful and joyful moments.

856. Make Sure Your Home Is Healthy: While paying attention to the aesthetics of your home, take some time to investigate whether or not your home is healthy. An unhealthy home can contribute to your infertility. Is there mold or mildew in your home? Have an air quality test done in your home. Do you need to invest in a air purifier or HEPA filter system if you live in a high pollution area? Some studies hve suggested that the air inside most house is 5 to 10 times worse than the air outdoors. Does your heating system need to be professionally cleaned?

Do you have professional lawn care services that might be bringing lots of pesticides and chemicals into your life? Do you live in an older home that could still harbor lead paint, asbestos or arsenic? Do you have cabinets, paneling, plywood, particle board, carpets or furniture made with volatile organic compounds (VOCS)? Are the carpets in your home full of chemicals that emit VOCS?

Do you have moth balls in your home that contain the chemical paradichlorobenzene? Is there lead in your plumbing fixtures?
Do you use air fresheners that contain ethylene-based glycol ethers and terpenes? Could you have radon in your home or a carbon monoxide leak coming from a furnace, generator, or appliances? Be aware of the chemicals that you bring into your home and start using natural cleaners that are non-toxic or even make your own homemade cleaning products. Filter your tap water, use a vacuum cleaner with a HEPA filter to get as much dust as possible, and change your furnace filter often.

857. Bring Nature Indoors: Did you know that just touching a houseplant prompts a relaxing response in the brain? Create an indoor herb garden. Put plants all around your house. Buy yourself flowers every week. Note: if you have pets, do not bring in plants that are toxic and could hurt or kill them. If you have pets, you may want to consider a small greenhouse that your animals do not have access to.

858. Healthy Scents: No, this is not the time to buy air fresheners or any other type of scent that is not natural and could bring toxins into your environment, but you might want to consider bringing natural healthy scents into your home. Simmer orange peels, cloves, dried lavender, apple peels and cinnamon over the stove. Consider natural essential oils and grow fragrant herbs on your windowsill, such as rosemary.

859. Bring In The Pillows: Create comfort whenever you can.

860. Make Music Available: Get an iPod or even an old-fashioned stereo and set it up in the living room. When you are doing chores or cooking or put on some CDs. Make your home a place where music is readily available and accessible.

861. Tap Into The Power of Words: Think about what words, sayings or quotes you can use to decorate your home and lift your spirits each day. Or stencil your favorite quotes on a wall or on furniture. How about creating a wall of great quotes in a hallway or bathroom?

862. Welcome Some Water: Set up a plug-in tabletop fountain, buy a fish tank and fill it with beautiful fish and aquatic plants, hang photographs of the ocean or a beautiful lake. The sound of water can lower heart rates and stress levels. Studies have shown that just looking at a picture of water can induce feelings of relaxation.

863. Make Your Bedroom Conducive To A Good Night's Sleep: Getting a good night's sleep is key right now, so make sure your room is as dark as possible and no light is creeping into your bedroom at night. Get shade darkeners, heavy curtains, and unplug all electronics.

864. Be Yourself: Do you feel authentic in your home? Or is it set up to impress others? Is it decorated in a way that is true to who you are? Or does your home look like someone other than you should live there? Make your home a place that is authentically you.

865. Display It: A favorite doll, a momento from a great trip, your collection of seashells from a walk on the beach. If you have items that make you happy, and bring up feelings of peace from times gone by, put them out where you can see them. On my kitchen counter, I have items from my beach vacations that mean so much to me.

866. Make Your Workspace Pleasurable Too: While you may not be able to say goodbye to your annoying boss, you may be able to put a saying or a quote on your desk at work that gives you a measure of joy and peace.

867. Display Reminders of the Beautiful Relationships In Your Life: A gift from someone you love, a blanket your Mom made you, a loving card from a friend. Frame and display cards and letters from friends and family. How much happier our environments would be if we hung our cards instead of putting them away in drawers. How about making a collage of all your favorite cards from different times in your life?

868. Visualize Your Way To Your Baby

Here are some visualization exercises you can do to enhance your fertility:

See yourself standing in a field of colorful flowers. The flowers are opening and blooming, just as your body is blooming. See flowers blooming from your vaginal area as flowers continue to open all around you. You are a flowering blossom, part of the earth's beautiful eco-system, and blooming is happening all around you.

869. See light healing all your organs. It is entering and healing your uterus. The light is entering your liver and clearing your liver of all anger. The light is now entering your adrenal glands and giving all your glands energy and love. The light is shining into your stomach and taking away any nervous tension or stress that once lived there. The light is going into your head, your neck and your chest. Feel how good it is. See the light working its way through your body. It enters your chest and you can breath. It enters your ovaries and they can do what they are meant to do. The light travels through your body healing and soothing every part of your body.

870. See yourself walking hand-in-hand with your child. Look at your child's hands. Touch your hand, and imagine how it will feel when your child touches your hand.

871. Visualize walking into your baby's nursery and looking into a crib and picking up your beautiful baby. What do the windows look like in your baby's room? What type of bedding did you choose for your baby's crib? Imagine lifting your baby from the crib and sitting in a rocking chair. Ah, it feels so good to sit and rock your baby. Let yourself feel the peace and contentment of holding and rocking your baby.

872. See your husband/parter's sperm traveling up your vagina, meeting your egg, connecting, and then exploding with new life. See the embryo implant itself firmly into your uterus. See it growing into your baby.

873. Picture your ovaries turning and children jumping out from your ovaries.

874. It is the day of your child's wedding. Can you see yourself there? What are you wearing? See your child walking down the aisle. Your eyes are bright with happiness and you cannot stop smiling. Envision dancing with your child at the reception. Close your eyes and listen to a song you would like played at your child's wedding.

875. It is the day your baby is born. The nurse has just handed you your baby. Feel it. For one moment, let yourself experience the emotions you are going to feel. Picture it as if it already happened.

876. Look down at your stomach. You are pregnant. Say it out loud: I am pregnant. I am pregnant.' Pat your stomach. Doesn't it feel great to be pregnant? Tell your stomach you love it. Tell your baby you love him or her. Sit down and feel what it is like to be pregnant.

877. Imagine the sun shining directly on your vagina and healing everything within you.

878. **Fertility Affirmations:** Words have power. Words can help heal the body. Words can provide your heart with hope. Saying, writing, singing, and reading affirmations everyday can lift your mood and help you physically manifest what you most want. Go ahead, begin affirming out loud that yes, you are going to have a baby! Yes, your dream of becoming a mother is going to come true!

Doing affirmations will give you a chance to take conscious control of your thoughts. No longer will negative thoughts have free rein to take over and demoralize you. You deserve to hear affirmations that positively announce the arrival of your baby.

Affirmations will help you combat the negativity, frustration and fear that often accompany infertility. They will give you a powerful way to tap into joyful, hopeful emotions that you deserve to feel as you walk down this exciting life path.

Affirmations can slowly transform a subconscious who may have given up, into a subconscious that really and truly believes a baby will be arriving soon. Your body then can easily move into a state of hope and belief. A body that believes will act accordingly, because it knows that a wonderful guest is about to arrive.

As you say your affirmations, breath them, feel them, visualize them coming true. Let them sink so deep into your body that your very essence soaks them in as if watching a dream come true.

Repeat your affirmations as much as possible. Speak them, write them, sing them, turn them into poems, repeat and do it all again. Write and speak them, even if you do not believe them at first.

By affirming your baby's arrival, you are emitting positive energy into the world—an energy working towards your goal, not against it.

When you say out loud, "I can and will have a baby" you are using the energy of words to manifest what you most want.

Some ways to state your affirmations include:

879. Write your affirmations and post them on a mirror or wall that you can look at each morning as you get ready for your day ahead.

880. Get a notebook and spend five to ten minutes a day writing your affirmations. As you write, speak the words out loud.

881. Record yourself saying your affirmations, either on your phone, iPod of CD, and listen to them when you take a walk or simply are doing chores around the house.

882. Listen to a recording of your affirmations and visualize what you are saying coming true as you listen to them. You can add background music if that makes the affirmations more powerful to you.

883. Choose one or two affirmations that are easy to say and say them when you wake up each morning. They could be something simple like: 'I am ready to have a baby' or 'My baby is arriving soon.'

884. Create a piece of art or draw a picture that includes one or two affirmations that are important and meaningful to you.

885. Hang a chalkboard and write your affirmations daily. If you can, put the chalkboard in a place where you see it often.

886. Buy a calendar or an appointment book and write affirmations in each date. Below are affirmations that you can do daily. Choose the ones that strike you most powerfully and that you most feel your body needs to hear often. Think about what negative beliefs you hold about your fertility that need to be replaced with positive, hopeful words.

- I trust my body can give me a baby.

- I give myself permission to have a baby.

- I grant myself the power to have a baby.

- My body is making a baby right now.

- I am ready to have a baby.

- I am ready to be pregnant.

- I am ready to be a mother.

- I am good enough to be a mother.

- I now welcome my baby.

- My body is creating lots of healthy eggs today.

- I will get pregnant today.

- My embryos are successfully implanted in my uterus and my baby is now on the way to me.

- I am an amazing mother about to have an amazing baby!

- I enjoy bringing new life into the world.

- My pregnancy is perfect.

- I agree to have a baby.

- Love surrounds me as I welcome my baby.

- I am ready, willing and able to get pregnant.

- I have the power in my body and heart to create a baby.

- Hip, hip hooray there is joy in my day!

- Its okay to get pregnant.

- My body is fertile and healthy

- I am pregnant with a beautiful, healthy baby

- My body knows how to get pregnant and care for my baby.

- I trust in my ability to give birth to a baby.

- I know how to meet the needs of my baby and myself

- Today, I will allow myself to get pregnant.

- I am allowing myself to become a mother.

- I feel relaxed and confident about my pregnancy.

- The birth experience will be wonderful for me and my baby.

- I am going to deliver a happy, healthy baby.

- I can see myself playing with my beautiful baby.

- My body is beautifully nourishing my baby.

- I conceive my baby with love, I carry my baby with love, I deliver my baby with love, and I welcome my baby with love.

- My body is a healthy perfect place for my baby to grow.

- I love getting pregnant.

- I love being ripe and fertile.

- I love being ready to welcome my baby.

- Every part of me is ready to have a baby.

- My body is fertile and full of healthy babies.

- My eggs are fertile, ripe and healthy.

- My womb is strong and fertile.

- I am completely deserving of a baby.

- My body knows how to get pregnant and carry my baby full-term

- Everything and everyone around me is helping me get pregnant

- My hormones are balanced and working just as they should

- My liver, ovaries and adrenal glands are strong and healthy

- I am ready to welcome my baby

- This is the perfect time and perfect age for me to have a baby

- I am strong enough to have a baby

- My uterus is safe and strong

- My ovaries are powerful, strong and ready

- I am worthy of having a child

- I accept the miracle of birth into my life

- I am part of the natural birth cycle

- I will successfully conceive and give birth to a baby

- I will have a baby, I will have a baby, I will have a baby

- My body says it is okay to have a baby

- My body has agreed to have a baby

- I am ready to have a baby

- I welcome my baby into my life

- It is safe for my baby to be born

- There is nothing blocking me from having a baby

- I am fertile

- I am full of hope and confidence that soon I will become a mother

- My baby is arriving soon

- I accept my right to be a mother

- Nothing from my past can hurt me anymore

- I am safe and I am loved.

- My mind, body and emotions are healed so I can now have a baby

- Having a baby is fun and relaxing

- My body says yes to having a baby!

- I deserve to be a mother

- I am going to be a great Mom

- My body has everything it needs to conceive a healthy baby

- I am healthy and ready to conceive

- I am able to receive and give birth to a baby

- Love and goodness follow me daily

- I am able to carry a pregnancy full-term

- I am able to conceive a child

- I am able to carry a pregnancy full-term and give birth to a healthy baby

- I am pregnant

- My body is ready, willing and able to be pregnant

- I can give birth whenever I choose

- Giving birth is easy for me

- Giving birth is safe for me

- I am capable of being a mother

- Nothing in my past prevents me from being a mother

- I give myself permission to be pregnant

- I am strong and able to conceive a baby

- My body is ready to lovingly produce a baby

- My ovaries are good and strong

- My ovaries are now making lots of healthy eggs!

- My baby is on the way to me

- I am a mother

- I am giving birth. I am holding life in my arms

- I can carry my baby for nine months

- Every part of my body is ripe for the birth and creation process.

- I am ripe and ready to conceive

- I am receiving my baby right now.

- I am holding my baby.

- I am ready to receive a baby.

- I am ready to give birth.

- I give myself permission to get pregnant.

- I grant myself the power to get pregnant.

- I have permission to be a mother.

- It is safe for me to have a baby

- It is safe for me to become a mother

- I have permission to have a baby

- My body has the power to conceive and give birth to a child

- I am deserving of a child

- I deserve a baby

- My vagina, ovaries, kidney and liver are strong and healthy

- I welcome my baby

- My body is helping me get pregnant

- My body is ready to have a baby

- My womb is ready to receive a baby

888. **Your Personal Fertility Vision Statement:** A personal vision statement is something you can read, record and listen to each day. When you listen, visualize what is being said so it can sink deep into your subconscious. Be sure to fill in your name.

889. **Here is your personal vision statement:**

It is a bright, warm, sunny morning and you are feeling really good. You walk outside, take a deep breath of fresh air, raise your arms to the sky and say thank you, thank you, thank you for my baby.

That's right, YOUR NAME_____, having a baby is easy for you. Your body and mind are ready, willing and VERY able to have a baby.

You smile, because being vibrantly healthy and super fertile feels good.

Really good actually.

You know on a very deep level that having a baby is good and right for you. You deserve this baby. You are completely and totally worthy of having a baby.

You are capable of conceiving a baby, carrying a baby for nine months and giving birth, in the healthiest, safest, most wonderful way possible.

That's right, you are worthy of having children.

Because you ate so many healthy green vegetables, let go of the toxins in your body, and said goodbye to all the trauma, anger and sadness in your cells, you are now able to give birth to a baby whenever you choose.

That's right: you can have a baby whenever you want to. Today, next week, next month, whenever you choose. Your body has the power to conceive and give birth to a baby whenever you want it to.

You can see yourself smiling and holding your new baby. You see yourself kissing your baby and feeling so thankful that your baby has arrived.

You look in the mirror and smile, because being a mother feels right to you.

Your baby is here. You are fertile. You are super fertile today! You are actually over-the-top fertile right now! You are creating super healthy eggs this minute.

That's right: your dear sweet ovaries are right now producing ripe, rich, healthy eggs. Feel how strong and good your eggs are!

Your body now has everything it needs to get pregnant. All the organs in your body are working at maximum capacity to help you get pregnant. Your liver has let go of anger and is now balanced and calm. Your kidneys have let go of sadness and are happy now.

Nothing in your past can block you from conceiving and giving birth. You forgive those who hurt you. You released all anger and sadness. You have let go of all the bad memories, sad events, and traumas in your life. Only happiness lives in your cells now.

Love and happiness flow through your body now. Love flows into your heart.

That's right, there is immense power in your heart to have a baby.

You have permission to have a baby. You have permission to conceive. You have permission to enjoy a safe and successful pregnancy. You are ready to give birth.

Your hurt is gone. Your anger is gone. Your fear is gone. You are safe.

That's right, you feel safe all the time. Safer than you ever felt before. You know it is safe for you to get pregnant and safe for you to give birth and safe for you to be a mother. Life is safe. Motherhood is safe. Having children is safe. Everything is safe.
You feel safe all the time, because you know that having a baby is safe for you.

All fears and pain from your childhood are gone. All your anxiety is gone. All your frustration is gone.

You laugh and feel happy.

That's right, you laugh a lot lately, because feeling so healthy and fertile feels good.

Really good actually. Life is so good!

Your body is now full of pure and clean energy. Your bowels are clean and you eliminate easily. Your blood sugar levels are stable. Your hormones are balanced and communicate well with one another. Your pituitary gland, adrenal gland, thyroid and pancreas are healthy and balanced. Blood flows easily to your uterus.

Oxygen flows easily to your ovaries. Your uterine lining is strong. Your vagina is open and ready to receive. Your ovaries are making lots of healthy eggs.

That's right, your ovaries are now making strong, viable healthy eggs that make it easy for you to conceive and give birth.

You now flow with life. You feel comfortable asserting your will. You let your authentic voice be heard. You welcome your real self. You respect yourself. You no longer feel shame or guilt. You honor and express all your feelings. You creativity express yourself, as having a baby is a creative expression you fully allow yourself.

You smile and feel relaxed.

You feel relaxed a lot lately. You slept so good last night. You sleep good every night.

That's right, you are relaxed and sleeping well because you know everything is going to be okay.

It is okay for you to get pregnant and have lots of babies.

You smile, because you always knew you would get pregnant.

That's right. You knew that infertility was just a temporary condition. You knew you would heal and be fertile. You always said, "I will get pregnant soon" and you were right.

You have already let yourself receive a baby. Your womb is a warm, welcoming place for your babies.

You are strong enough to receive and hold your baby.

Nothing in your past can hold you back having the children you desire. You deserve this! Go ahead. Let yourself have this. Let yourself have your babies!

You, my darling, are part of the world's unstoppable, undefeatable, always victorious birth cycle. See that flower blooming—you are part of that bloom. See that tree sprouting new leaves—you are part of that sprouting! You are part of life's beautiful birth cycle. You have everything you need within you to give birth to a baby, just like all the other living beings on the planet.

You got it kid! You do! Your dream of being a mother is now coming true. You are allowed to have a baby. It is good and right and okay for you to have a baby. It is safe for you to be a mother.

That's right—you are meant to have a baby. Things are working out for you, just as you hoped they would.

It feels right and good to receive your baby. Your body feels good doing this. Giving birth is fun. Being a mother is fun. Getting pregnant is fun.

Go ahead and have a baby! It is okay! You have given yourself permission! Every part of your body has agreed to help you conceive and give birth.

Getting pregnant is easy for you.

Go ahead, today is the day you can conceive your beautiful baby.

Then do it again whenever you want too, because getting pregnant and having children is easy, safe and fun for someone like you.

890. **The Emotion of Deserving:** Emotionally, it is important to root out every single thought that you may possibly hold about not deserving a baby. If you are a person who s feels undeserving of good things, you might on some level not feel you are worthy of receiving a baby. Many people say they want something, but on some level, they don't really think they deserve it.

Because of this deep subconscious belief, they prevent themselves from actually attaining what they want because a part of them simply doesn't think they deserve to get it.

That subconscious feeling of not being worthy can lead a person to make the wrong choices, sabotage efforts, derail progress, to confirm the notion that they are not worthy of attaining their desire.

Not feeling deserving is a dangerous emotion—like harboring a spy who pretends to be on your side, but is actually working against you. You need to convince every part of your body that yes, you deserve a baby.

All your thoughts and feelings of not being deserving must be eliminated. If you think you are unworthy of having a baby, you may not put forth all the effort needed to achieve your aim. A person who feels undeserving may "prick their own balloon" sabotaging their efforts. If you think you don't deserve something, you may never let yourself attain what you want. How? By allowing your subconscious to make choices that prevent you from reaching your goal.

If you can get to the point where you truly believe you deserve something, you will do things, welcome things, invite things, and make choices, that improve your chances of getting what you rightfully feel you deserve.

Write down these words: 'I deserve a baby.' Now write down whatever comes up--do not overthink it or analyze it--just write down your response. Now do it again. Write: 'I deserve a baby.' Do not analyze what you write, just let whatever is within you bubble up.

Now, what did you find out? Does your subconconscious truly think you deserve a baby? It is important to know exactly what your subconscious thinks about you deserving a child. Remember--you are a living being and with that, you were born deserving the right to procreate if you choose. It is a right, inherent from the moment you were born.

Here is something to cut out and read daily. Say these words out loud. Shout them, put them deep in your heart, whisper them at your most difficult moments, sing them, visualize them, repeat them over and over, write them, type them, say them over again, hang them in places you can see daily.

• I deserve to have a baby.

- I deserve to be pregnant.
- I am good enough to be pregnant.
- I am ready to receive the gift of a baby.
- I give myself permission to become pregnant.
- I grant myself the power to become pregnant.
- I am worthy of having a baby.
- I deserve to have this work out.
- I deserve to give birth.
- My body deserves to be happy and healthy.
- I deserve to be a mother.
- I deserve to love a baby and be loved in return.
- I deserve good things.
- I am a living being who deserves to able to bring life from my body, just like that tree outside or that flower or an ant.
- My body deserves and wants to have a baby.
- I deserve a child.
- I deserve to be a mother.
- I am good enough to be a mother.
- I am worthy of holding my child in my arms.

Remember--feeling deserving does not mean you are vain, egotistical, selfish, spoiled, or somehow a bad person. Feeling deserving means you understand that as a human being, you are gifted with some basic rights—and that you don't have to be perfect to enjoy some of the pleasures and rewards that come with being a human.

Feeling deserving means that regardless of past mistakes, you sense that as a human being, being happy is something you have a right to. So repeat after me: I deserve to have a baby...I deserve to have a baby...

891. **Start Living Authentically:** An often overlooked part of healing from infertility is living your life through your authentic original self.

Having a baby is a very natural, authentic process, and if you have buttoned up yourself to the point that doing anything real and authentic is absent, you may need to tap back in and welcome your true self.

You need to reunite with your true self so that you can feel completely at home in your body.

Feeling comfortable in your own skin and feeling at home in your body will help release inner reserves of energy, nourishment and peace that could help heal your infertility.

You have the right to embrace and welcome your original authentic self—even if you have ignored her for a very long time.

The authentic self is the 'you' at core of who you really are, not the 'you' people have told you that you are suppose to be.

Due to feeling shamed, judged or rejected, many women live their life through fake, imposter personalities because their true self was never valued or accepted.

The original self is buried—this beautiful, wise, helpful part of ourselves—is left dormant and ignored.

She deserves better. You deserve better.

Starting today, listen to your real self. Let her speak. Pay attention to what she wants and needs.

The false self is stiff. She is not free or real. She lives her life in a defensive position always ready to protect herself from attack, judgment or rejection.

This results in a feeling of constant stress and a tightness that does not allow the body to flow naturally as it was meant to flow.

Starting now, do what comes naturally. Eat, breath, and live in a way that feels natural.

Stop being a robot trying to please others.

Get out of your head and into your heart.

Give yourself the freedom to be yourself.

Say goodbye to the imposter personalities that smother your true self.

Let your true self out! Let her breath! Give her what she wants!

Allow real connection with others. Stop living in a way that only allows artificial forms of connection and disconnects you from the natural world.

Ask yourself: what makes my soul happy and content? What am I truly drawn to?

Do one thing a day that puts you back in touch with your heart. Listen to the little voice in back of your mind. What is she telling you? Be aware of your true likes and dislikes.

Start living in a way that lets you to be comfortable in your own skin.

Let the real you come out and play.

Have you dimmed your inner light because you are afraid for people to see the real you?

Turn on your light! Let it shine!

Think back: who were you before IT happened? The IT being any event, person or experience that withered you a bit, stole your confidence, made you doubt yourself, broke your heart. What were you like?
Are there parts of your personality that are dormant because you are too afraid to let them out again? What were you like as a child? Does your personality today resemble who you were or are you completely different? Are you stuffing the real you to please everyone else? Stop stuffing and stop trying to please. As Anais Nin says, "and the day came when the risk to remain tight in a bud was more painful than the risk it took to blossom." Take the risk to blossom. Shake off the shame. Let go of the tightness within. Reveal your authentic self. Be 'her' as much as possible.Welcome back the parts of you that were shamed into hiding. Let them talk again! Express again! Let them be themselves again. Welcome back the real you.

Do more of whatever makes you feel alive and joyful. Be aware of your true feelings and preferences. What do you really want to wear? Who do you really want to spend time with?

Start living fully as your real self wants to live.

Stop hiding.

Move to your own rhythm, your own sense of selfhood.

Say yes only when you want to say yes to.

Stop judging yourself. Embrace your authentic ideas, values and personality traits.

Trust your instincts. Define your own values and youw own reality. Follow your intuition.

Your body will feel better and so will you.

892. **Welcoming Your Mother Within**: Within you lies a mother waiting for the moment when she can step forward and assume her rightly role. In many ways, you are probably already stepping forward into the role of a mother by the way you live your life. You have most likely done many things that demonstrate the maternal part of you. It is likely that you already have had the experience of mothering yourself and those around you. So Mom, let it show—you know you are already living and breathing this role that is rightfully yours.

Here are some ways to get in touch with your inner mother:

893. Begin today to see yourself as a mother. When you look in the mirror, remind yourself that yes, you are a mother, and it is only a matter of time before your children physically manifest themselves. Say aloud: I am a Mom. Picture being called 'Mom' or write: I am a Mom.

894. See yourself surrounded by children. They are smiling. They like you. They like to be with you. Visualize yourself surrounded by children often. Picture yourself enjoying your children, talking with them, playing, and doing things you know come naturally to you. When you picture yourself with your children, visualize it authentically—if you hate to bake, don't try to conjure up an image of yourself baking. Maybe you would rather be racing your children down the beach instead, or teaching them to use a hammer or repairing a fence together.

Maybe you love to read, and reading to your children is something you will cherish. Or maybe you want to put on some roller blades and coast down some trails with them. There are a million different ways a million different mothers enjoy their children.

895. Write down all the qualities you already have that you associate with being a mother. Examples can include: being responsible, kind, tender, generous, strong, ingenius, creative, courageous, honest, a hard worker, loving, understanding, gentle, funny, fun-loving, responsible, resourceful, directed, nurturing, a leader, active, empathetic, self-sacrificing, playful, self-disciplined, fun.

896. Write down all the ways you currently mother yourself and others. Examples: You bring goodies into work for your co-workers. You write cards to friends and family on a regular basis. You enjoy buying presents for others. You are always ready to help in time of crisis. You enjoy cooking for family and friends. You love planning surprise parties. You are a good listener. You are able to comfort others when needed. You work very hard. You donate your time, money or energy to charity. You enjoy giving massages or foot rubs. You are a go-getter and not afraid to take on challenges that frighten others. You are dependable, a leader, and very competent, so that your boss and others at work can always rely on you.

You go the extra mile in almost everything you do. You allow others the space and comfort to just be themselves. You are honest with yourself and others. You nurture others and give them the confidence and strength to grow.

897. Do you sometimes have a 'motherly instinct'? If so, how do you manifest it? Example: You love your pets and try to keep them safe.

898. Make a collage with a picture of yourself and pictures of all the ways you currently mother yourself and others. You can include pictures of yourself with nephews and nieces, cousins, friends and others. Also include pictures of yourself doing things you love that require contributing either at work, toward a charity or in some form in your life.

899. Make a list of all the ways you look forward to nurturing your future children.

900. Write a letter to your inner mother, and thank her all the ways she is ready to have a baby.

901. Hitting Bottom: There are moments in infertility that are so painful, that trying to give advice about how to cope with them almost seems disrespectful.

So I will apologize right now for even attempting to give advice on how to get through moments so devastating that there is really no solace.

The pain of not conceiving is not something to be taken lightly, or something that some best-ten-tips list can cure.

I have suffered that kind of pain. Pain so raw and disappointing, and so completely upsetting to life's balance, that any advice given on how to deal with it can feel trite and disrespectful.

Infertility can attack the core of a woman's intrinsic and basic sense of what is natural and right. When having a baby does not occur naturally, it can rock to the core the way a woman feels about her life in general.

For a woman who desires children, not being able to reproduce can sting like a bloody violation of one of the most basic human rights.

So in your most painful moments, remember this: if you desire to be a mother more than anything, you will find a way to be a parent, either biologically or through adoption.

Your misery will fuel you to do whatever you need to do to become a parent. Your intense pain may be the reason you agree to undergo yet another IVF, and it may be that one more try that wins you the baby of your dreams.

Or that misery may push you to adopt an adorable baby and still try for a biological child.

All I know is no one wants to stay in the stalemate of misery indefinitely, and if you can't stand this feeling, then be glad for a moment, because that horrible feeling will push you to do things, try things, continue things, open yourself up to things, and never give up on things that could very well bring the child of your dreams into your life...as long as you don't give up and get stuck in the misery.

Please understand that anyone so desperately sad about not having a child is desperately needed in this world. You are needed in this world.

A person who is a lover of children is a treasure. This world desperately needs people who want to parent and who love children, and will do anything for that privilege and responsibility. This world needs people who feel that children are a sacred trust, worth all the sacrifices, and not a burden.

And it isn't fair that you have to wait so long for that child you want.

Your attitude toward having children is very different from those who see children as annoying nuisances who do nothing but drop crumbs on the floor, rather than the sacred gift they are.

For that kind of pain, you deserve an applause, a standing ovation, a huge golden trophy, a million hugs. I have lived through the wretchedness of feeling you are being robbed from the life and family experience you always imagined yourself having.

I have walked that road of bitterness, anger and frustration so intense that nothing I have ever experienced compared to the utter misery of not being able to conceive and bear a child.

Having a child is a right every woman is born with, and to not be able to fulfill this inherited natural human right is beyond painful and grueling. When I reached my lowest points of misery, I sobbed without shame on the steps of an old run down donut shop in an ailing, decrepit town.

On another occasion, after learning I was not pregnant, I cried so much that my neighbors overheard me and were convinced my husband was beating me.

Once, I was so distraught after an IVF that didn't work, I left 12 messages on the voice mail of my nursing team at the clinic asking question after question about what might have gone wrong. So I'm assuming you will be a lot saner in your darkest moments than I was. But if you are not, that is okay and completely understandable too. You will find a way to survive this, thrive and fulfill your need to love and care for children. Just remember a few things:

902. Keep Believing: Never stop believing that something good is about to happen. The ability to keep hope alive and keep a believing attitude even during the darkest moments can motivate you to keep trying.

Never stop seeing and visualizing that baby you long to hold. Picture it, envision it, talk to it, believe that little sweet human is coming. Hold on to hope even when it looks like you should give up. Act as if it already happened. Each morning, step outside your door, raise your hands to the sky and say, "I am ready to receive a baby" or "thank you. I am ready to receive my baby." When you wake up each morning, whisper, "I am pregnant." When you get out of bed, walk like you are pregnant, act like you are pregnant, and repeat the words, "I am pregnant. I am pregnant."

903. Use Your Anguish To Generate Change: Nothing motivates a person to action like intense emotional pain. When the pain is so bad you can't stand it, you will also be hitting a powerful emotional point: Stay open. Answers can come when you are in this type of pain. You may be willing to go the extra mile that you were unwilling to go before.

Your pain can be the motor that keeps you going--so as bad as it feels, don't hate it. Great revolutions and profound historical changes have often been propelled by those in so much pain, they had no choice but to force change and make life better. Your pain will force change too. You will find a way to fill that vacuum inside you--as long as you don't let the pain crush you, stop you, or submerge you into a helpless pit.

When you are in that kind of pain, you will be faced with two choices--either you can fall into a pit of despair and drown, or you can kick and scream and demand that something different happen.

Every day, make one choice that will move you forward and bring you one step closer to your dream. Choose action over inaction. That way you won't be permanently stuck in the pit of despair.

904. When You Have Reached What Seems Like A Dead End, Take An Unexpected Turn in the Road: Go left. Go right. Start over and do it again. Close your eyes and walk backwards. Try to think about getting pregnant in new ways, analyzing the situation from various perspectives. Picture yourself sitting at a table with the world's greatest minds: what advice would they give you about your infertility? Be open to the ideas that come. Pretend someone else is in your situation, and ask yourself: what would your inner, say, Oprah Winfrey, do in this instance? Or your inner Eleanor Roosevelt? What advice does your inner Einstein have for you? How about Dr. Phil or Ghandi?

905. Go To A Trauma Release Specialist: Your body needs to release all the pain and trauma that can result from enduring infertility. Find a chiropractor, kinesiologist or myofascial release expert in your area who specializes in body work or trauma release. Write a list or a paragraph of what you have gone through and give it to the trauma release practitioner. Let them work on releasing whatever traumas are lodged in your body. By doing this, you will be freeing up some energy so you have the stamina it takes to continue infertility treatments.

906. Read Inspirational Books and Listen to Inspiring Music: Put your mind's focus on what inspires and uplifts you. Bring hopeful music and books into your life. Fertilize your soul with positive words.

907. Always Remember that During Life's Darkest Moments, The Sun Can Peek Through the Clouds: Today's heartbreak could end up being the chubby-cheeked twins keeping you up all night next year at this time.

908. Pain Can Destroy You or Motivate You to Win: Don't let your pain immobilize or debilitate you. Instead, use your pain to propel you to action. Let your pain be a motivator—not a destroyer. Use your pain to help you determine what is happening within your body. Then, let the pain of wanting a baby motivate you to make the changes necessary for your body to get stronger and better able to conceive a child.

909. Understand that Your Drive to Parent Will Find a Home in This World: An empty space does not stay empty forever. Voids find a way to be filled. Your fervent desire to be a parent will seek until that desire is filled in some way. You will be a mother. You will make it so. That empty space inside you will be filled. You will find a way.

910. Persist: When you hit bottom, resolve to try again and try again and yes, try again. Don't let even the most devastating cycle or news prevent you from saying: how about one more try?

911. Change Something or Stick with Something: Ask yourself: is there something in my journey through infertility that needs to be changed? Am I satisfied with my doctor and the clinic I am going to? Do I need to eat differently? Or, are you already doing lots of positive things that just need time to work and require that you persistently stick to doing them? Don't get stuck if change is needed and don't give up and grow impatientif you are already doing something right that will help you get pregnant.

912. Make a List of Every Dream or Goal You Achieved: Write down every goal you accomplished that required hard work, patience, effort and persistence. List every obstacle you overcame to achieve that dream. Refer to this list often as a reminder that dreams and much sought after goals really do come true. Remind yourself of how you have won in the past, and how you will win again in the future.

Use this list as a reminder that obstacles can be surmounted, and what seems impossible today can become tomorrow's reality.

913. Find Places to Put Your Pain: Swim, write in a journal, paint. Engage in creative ways to release your pain and disappointment. Give your pain a chance to escape your body. Buy a keyboard and invent original tunes. Sing whenever you can. Write stories about your fertility experience. Create a cartoon or fairy tale about your journey to having a baby—and give it a happy ending! Dance your pain away. Write your pain away. Sing your pain away. Look for ways to physically expulse your stress, frustration and pain.

914. Participate in the Process of Creation So That You Experience That Creating Something is Possible For You: As you walk this road in creating a baby, allow yourself to experience the creation process that occurs every day in our world. Let your body feel the relief and joy that comes with creating, whether it is making a sculpture with pie dough or growing a plant in your kitchen. Create a new recipe, create a piece of art, create a garden, create a dollhouse, make something out of fabric. Do things that remind your inner self that you have the ability to create. Keep a journal titled: What I Created Today and write about one thing you create each day.

915. Notice the Birth Process in the World Around You Each Day: Look around and notice the birth process occurring in the world around you each day—and remind yourself that very soon you are going to be part of that beautiful process too.

Visit an animal shelter and spend time with kittens or puppies. Walk through a park and notice the cycle of life happening all around. Observe how weeds grow in the oddest, most difficult places. Watch how bugs and animals can reproduce in your home even when you don't want them too—and then feel your connection to this process as much as you can at this time.

916. Regardless of How Badly You Feel, Keep the Positive Words Flowing: Even in your darkest moments, continue to speak of hope. Never say: "I'll probably never get pregnant" or "Nothing works out for me" or "This is a big waste of time" or "I hate myself for this."

Keep affirming aloud to others and silently to yourself that yes, you will get pregnant....yes, you will have a baby...yes, you will conceive and deliver a beautiful baby.

Even when you are feeling devastated and expressing your sadness to a friend or family member, make sure all your conversations include statements like: "as hard as this is, I know deep in my heart I will have a baby soon" or "I really believe my body is healing and I am about to conceive a child" or "a year from now, I'm going to be holding my baby."

917. Stay Close To Positive People: Keep close in touch with positive people, and let their positive words sink deep into every part of your consciousness.

918. Become Best Friends With Your Body: Start enjoying a close, loving friendship with your body. Talk lovingly to your body each day. Let your body know you have complete confidence in its ability to conceive and give birth. Say: "I love you body." Treat your body with kindness. See the efforts your body is making and praise it. Get optimistic with your body! Tell your body that it is strong, it is capable, and all your organs are doing a great job of getting ready to be pregnant. Let your ovaries know you love them and you have full faith in their ability to create and release healthy eggs. Say I love you to your uterus every day. Let your thyroid gland know you love it and believe it can sustain and nurture you. Treat your body as you would a beloved best friend.

919. Prayer: For me, the most powerful antedote to my pain was prayer. During my rock bottom moments, it was only through prayer that I was able to find strength and hope.

During my most hopeless moments, it was only my hope that God would help me have the babies I so long for that carried me through and enabled me to keep going.

Without the privilege of being able to pray to God, I would never have been able to endure the painful disappointments I experienced during my infertility treatments. If not for prayer, I would not have had the strength to continue on. Sometimes, for me, the greatest and sometimes only antidote to my pain was prayer.

920. Help Others: When you hit bottom, set out to help another person who is going through a tough time too. Make it your goal to spread hope to someone who needs hope as badly as you do. Wanting a child is, in part, a desire to give to and love someone outside yourself on a permanent basis. As you await the arrival of your child, keep in mind the other people in this world who need your love. Yes, you deserve a child to love and nothing can replace that, but while you wait, think about where your love is needed in this world and who you can help with all the love inside you.

921. Let Yourself Fall Apart and Then Get Up Again: When you reach a crisis point and are overwhelmed with grief, let yourself fall apart but then, get up and begin trying again. Infertility can be a wrenching experience and you have the right to mourn...so mourn...but at a certain point, get up and try again.

922. Start A 'Reason to Hope' Journal: Every day, find reasons to hope and write them down. Be on the lookout for anything in your life, your world, your surroundings that give you a reason to hope. Open your eyes wide and find one hopeful and positive thing to write about. Any time you find a reason to hope, write it down.

923. Read Inspirational True-to-Life Stories of People Who Were Down and Out, but Somehow Managed to Turn Things Around: Soak your mind in true-to-life stories of miracles, of people who beat impossible odds and managed to overcome the challenges they faced. Read about people who are medical miracles and who somehow defied all the odds. Put so many impossible-but-came-true tales in your head that soon you won't see having a baby as something out of your reach at all.

924. Watch The Movie Rocky: Watch all of them. Then watch them again.

925. Make Sure to Eat Well, Sleep Well, and Do Everything in Your Power to Keep the Happy Chemicals in Your Brain Dancing: Work on keeping the chemicals in your body and brain as happy as possible. If you eat badly, the chemicals in your brain will work against you--making an already stressful situation more stressful.

When you eat healthy and get the rest you need, you are giving your brain and body the power it needs to support your emotional self. Think: lots of greens, some berries, nuts and seeds, early bedtime and light exercise. Make the chemicals in your body your ally.

926. Put Together a Strategy If You Don't Have One: Creating a step-by-step fertility plan will keep you focused and moving forward when you reach crisis points. Rather than immobilized by disappointment, knowing your next step, and the next step after that, will keep you moving forward towards your goal.

927. Remind Yourself That You Are One Tough Cookie: Repeat after me: I am one tough cookie, I am one tough cookie...I can do what it takes to get what I want...I can do what it takes to get my baby.

928. Say These Affirmations Each Day: When you are feeling down, write, type, sing, and speak these affirmations:

I am strong and able to conceive a baby.

My body is love and ready to love my baby.

My ovaries are making lots of healthy eggs!

My baby is on the way to me.

I am a mother. I give birth. I am holding life in my arms.

I receive my baby

I can carry my baby for nine months and then give birth.

Every part of my body is ready to be pregnant.

I am ripe and ready to conceive.

I am receiving my baby right now.

929. Remember, as a Woman on This Planet Earth, You Are Already A Mother--and Are Now Just Waiting to Manifest Your Motherhood in a Physical Sense Differently Than You've Expressed It Before: If you look after a family member's health, if you buy presents for someone else's children, if you care about the emotional well-being of your friends, if you bring goodies to work for your co-workers...if you give your money or time to a charity...if you care for a pet, if you really, really love someone...then you have already begun your journey as a mother on this planet earth.

One of the definitions of the word 'mother' is 'a creative source' and that, I am willing to bet, you already are. So manifesting a physical child is not a huge stretch for you. Remind yourself that you are already a mother and will soon give birth to your own baby that will continue your mothering experience.

Another definition of mother is "to watch over, nourish and protect maternally." Your maternal spirit, evidenced by your drive to be a mother, is already in action. Take your power as a maternal being and put it out into the world. Acknowledge that you are, and have always been, a mother. Feel a certain ripeness and centering in your stomach as you acknowledge that you are already a mother, just waiting to physical manifest your already existing motherhood.

930. Start Getting In the Habit of Taking Care of Living Things: Begin taking care of living things right now, as a way to prepare to care for your babies. Get a pet, plant a garden, commit to feeding the birds, deer or turkeys in your area. Practice nurturing living things. As you do this, say to yourself: "I care for living beings on this earth as I will soon care for my babies."

931. Create Personal Rituals That Strengthen You and Give You Hope: When I first began infertility treatments, I would play the theme to the movie "Rocky" and march around my living room as the song played, all the while imagining my ovaries churning and babies popping out.

Strange yes, and thankfully no one ever caught me in my marching mode, but this routine strengthened me and by the end of this exercise, I felt strong, ready and the possibility of having children felt very, very real to me. Choose a song to be your personal anthem and dance, march, do whatever your body calls you to do.

932. Spend at Least 15 minutes a Day Outdoors in the Sunshine Looking at Nature: Let the warmth and light of the sun lift your sadness. Look at greenery whenever you can.

933. Tend to Your Spiritual Self: Pray, help others, read a book that uplifts your spirit, memorize Bible verses, record your appreciation for even the littlest things in a 'big fat thank you' gratitude journal.

934. Keep Going: When you hit bottom and feel your worst, keep going-- to your appointments, for treatments--just keep going.

935. Act As If There Is No Doubt This Will All Work Out: Each day, do one thing that demonstrates in a complete and tangible way that you truly believe you will give birth to a baby soon. Start planning your Disney vacation that you will bring your children on in a few years. Sew play clothes, build a toy chest for all the toys that will be in your home soon.

936. **Remember Who You Are:** Even in your darkest moments, it is important to remind yourself of who you are. Your infertility is just a temporary condition that has the potential to be healed. It is not a definitive statement on who you are or what you are capable of experiencing.

You are:

937. Capable: You are capable. To get through the rigors of infertility, you must remind yourself that you are capable--capable of working hard to get what you most desire, capable of healing, capable of conceiving, capable of carrying a baby full-term. You are capable. Your body is capable. Your reproductive organs are capable. Remind yourself of all the times when you were capable enough to defeat difficult challenges in your life.

930. Deserving: You deserve a baby. You are VERY deserving of a baby. You deserve this to work out. You deserve to see your dreams come true. Your body deserves the pleasure of conceiving and giving birth to a baby. You deserve to hear 'yes you are pregnant' and nine months later, you deserve to hold your beautiful baby in your arms.

939. Positive: You are positive. Within you lives a positive voice who has the strength to stay positive even when things are difficult.

940. Hopeful: You are hopeful. You hope because you know you have many good reasons to hope. You hope because good things happen to millions of people every single day. You hope because the human body is strong and can heal even from the most terrible illnesses. You hope because you've seen others have good results from their efforts. You hope because something deep inside you knows it is okay to hope. You hope because you have faith. You hope because this has worked out for others before you. You hope because you know today's no can turn into tomorrow's yes. You hope because the birth process goes on millions and millions of times each day, in all kinds of conditions, in millions of places, to all kinds of different people, and one of these days, it very well could include you. You hope because the human body can heal.
You hope because you know infertility is a temporary condition that can be fixed and overcome.

941. Committed: You are committed. You are committed to your goal of having a baby. You are committed to doing whatever is necessary to bring your baby to life. You are committed to doing the work, asking the questions, putting in the time, and taking this journey step by step to get what you want. Your body is committed to becoming healthy and fertile. Your reproductive organs are committed to giving you a baby. You are so committed that you will do and learn and understand whatever it is you have to do and learn and understand to conceive and give birth to your baby.

942. Determined: You are determined. You will plow through to get what you want. You are so determined that you refuse to give up until you have what you want. Your dogged determination empowers you to surmount all obstacles.

You refuse to listen to the naysayors, the discouragers, the pessimists or anyone else who is not supportive of you. You will try again and try again and try again as many times as you need to try to attain your goal. You realize there will moments of pure discouragement, but you won't let these times stop you you from stepping forward toward your ultimate purpose. Call you stubborn. Call you unstoppable. Call you the most determined mother on earth—a quality your future children will cherish, because the determination that helped you get pregnant will also help you build a great life for your kids.

943. Curious: You are curious. You ask questions, research, investigate, read, and ask more questions again. You want to know why your body is having trouble getting pregnant and you are not afraid to look for the answers. Your curiosity will move you to search out the reasons behind what is happening to you.

944. Unstoppable: You are unstoppable. Repeat after me: I am unstoppable! I am unstoppable! I am an unstoppable mother-to-be!

945. Powerful: You are powerful. You have the power to believe, power to pray, power to persevere, power to heal, power to think positive thoughts, power to visualize.

946. Ready to Heal: You are ready to heal. Your body is ready to heal. Your hormones are healing and balanced. Everything in your body is healing. Regardless of whatever news you hear from the clinic today, your body is continually walking forward towards healing.

947. Steady: You are steady. Step by step, inch by inch, day by day: you steadily do the things needed to attain your goal. You keep your 'eye on the ball' and never forget your purpose. Steadily, you are becoming more and more fertile by the day.

.

948. Nurturing: You are nurturing to yourself during this time. You give your spirit what it needs to endure this. You do things that uplift and soothe your soul. You put yourself around nurturing people. You engage in nurturing activities. You know how to nurture yourself, and this is going to be very useful because soon you will be called upon to nurture your new baby.

949. Loving: You are loving. Love gives you an undefeatable power and strength. Fueled by love, nothing can stop you. What force is more potent and unstoppable than love? Absolutely nothing.

950. **Coping With Shots and Injections:** Enduring injections is part of the infertility process. The first time I did it, I worried about it all day. As the time came closer to the 'shot', I felt like I was trapped in some type of dreaded countdown. It never really became easy, I found ways that made it bearable and sometimes relatively painless.

Here are my best tips for coping with injections:

951. If your husband or someone else is giving you the injection, have something interesting that you can read sitting in front of you. For me, I put a beautiful book on bed and breakfast inns in front of me. The lovely blue cover on the book soothed my soul. It was pretty and sweet, and represented everything that getting an injection wasn't. Looking at it was an escape: I'm not about to get a shot...I am visiting a lovely bed and breakfast inn and about to have homemade blueberry muffins, jam and a cup of tea. Right before my husband would insert the needle, I would turn to a recipe in this book and start reading it. Somehow, doing this helped me get through the many nights (and years) of shots.

952. Put on a favorite song, some comforting music, or a real party song. Close your eyes and sing-along.

953. My opinion: Don't look. Especially if the shots scare you, it is best not to look. Close your eyes and look away.

954. I am an expulsive person. I like to talk and expulse my feelings. For me, it helped to exhale through my mouth a few breaths during the shot. Using my breathing as a release always helped me.

955. Open a candy bar or some favorite food and smell it, take a bite. Distraction works. A delicious chocolate, a song, a book—get your senses engaged in something else during the injection.

956. Remind yourself that the discomfort you might experience is going to be worth it. Give yourself something to look forward to when it is over.

957. **How To Protect A Cherished Pregnancy:** If you have had recurrent miscarriages, you might want to:

• Ask to have an infection screen of your vagina.

• Ask for a Vitamin D deficiency test.

• Ask for a mineral deficiency test.

• Get tested for antiphospholipid syndrome (APS) which causes blood clots to form. A doctor can treat this condition with a low dose of baby aspirin or injections of heparin, which is a blood thinner.

• Visit your dentist and make sure there are no infections in your teeth or gums.

• Let your doctor know if you have any chronic conditions, such as thyroid disease, epilepsy, lupus, or a family history of clotting disorders.

958. **Some Ways To Protect Your Baby and Prevent A Miscarriage Once You Are Pregnant:** First off, it needs to be said: sometimes you can prevent a miscarriage and sometimes you can't. Most of the time, you can't. If you do miscarry, please know it is not your fault. Nature does this more often than we realize. Even in past generations, many women suffered miscarriages they knew nothing about. There are some things you can do to protect your growing baby, but please be aware that it is not your fault in any way if a pregnancy does not continue. The pain, of course, is immeasurable and intense, and there are no words to gloss over the immense sense of injustice and sadness this awful loss brings.

Here are some things you can do to help maintain a healthy pregnancy:

959. Boost Your Progesterone Levels: Maintaining adequate progesterone levels is absolutely key when you are pregnant. Ask your doctor if progesterone is something you should take to reduce the risk of miscarriage. If you have miscarried before, you might want to request progesterone from your doctor. Progesterone plays a role in maintaining the uterine lining, and because of this, some researchers have theorized that low progesterone plays a role in causing miscarriage.

Taking Vitamins C and B, and minerals such as zinc and magnesium, can help the body produce progesterone. Foods that help raise progesterone levels include: walnuts, bananas, wild yams, spinach and kale. Pumpkin, watermelon, chickpeas and squash seeds, which are high in zinc.

Try to avoid getting yourself in a stressful 'fight of flight' situation, which tends to reduce progesterone levels. Avoid all foods and herbs that can increase levels of estrogen, such as dong quai, hops, lavender, licorice, tea tree oil, and red clover blossom.

960. Keep Your Thyroid Healthy: If you have had recurrent miscarriages, you may want to have your thyroid tested to be sure you are maintaining a TSH above 2.0. Foods that encourage a healthy thyroid include artichokes and pineapple, which offer natural sources of iodine. Other foods to help the thyroid include garlic, sunflower seeds and turkey, which are high in selenium, and flaxseed, that contain high levels of Omega 3. Copper and iron rich foods are also very important to thyroid function. These include cashews, leafy greens,and lean red meats. Avoid Bromide, a chemical found in fluoride and chlorine, that disrupts the endocrine system. Bromide can also be found in soft drinks, plastics and some hair dyes. Also avoid soy, which some health practitioners believe can weaken the thyroid.

961. Nurture Your Kidneys: In Chinese medicine, it is believed that if a woman has suffered a miscarriage, she needs to work on her strengthening her kidney Qi. Start by drinking lots of water. Try to avoid situations that bring up feelings of fear.

Eating deep red foods like red bell peppers, red grapes, cranberries and beets, that can help rebuild and replenish the kidneys. Blueberries and apples are also good for the kidney. Avoid fluoride, artificial sweeteners and fructose. Avoid root canals and exposure to toxic mold, along with pesticides and toxic cleaning products.

962. Be Aware Of Your Homocysteine Levels: High levels of homocysteine can be a threat to your growing baby. Homocysteine is a sulfar-containing amino acid that can cause your blood to clot more easily. Be sure your prenatal vitamin has adequate levels of B6, B12, and folic acid, because this combination of B vitamins has been shown to prevent miscarriages that are caused by high homocysteine levels.

963. Avoid Excessively Stressful and Sad Situations: As much as possible, try not put yourself in situations that bring up extreme and intense feelings of fear, stress or sadness.. Stress tremendously affects the hormonal stability within the body. Let yourself sleep more, relax and say no to increased responsibilities and work at this time.

Avoid people, situations and activities that bring up a strong 'fight or flight' response. Limit time spent in situations where you feel nervous, anxious and uncomfortable. Do not listen to sad music or watch movies that bring up feelings of grief. Deep breath and give yourself permission to relax. Never underestimate how powerfully grief, sadness and toxic connections with others can impact your hormones.

964. Keep Your Hormones Stable: Keep your blood sugar levels stable, eat lots of leafy greens, don't exhaust your adrenal glands through stress or lack of rest. Foods that help balance hormones include olive oil and berries. Avoid white flour products, sugar, caffeine and alcohol.

965. Make Spinach Your Best Friend: Eat lots of spinach, it offers a rich form of iron that is needed for healthy cellular division.

966. Find Out If You Have Celiac Disease or Are Gluten Intolerant: Gluten, found in rye, wheat or barley, has been known to cause miscarriage in those who are allergic.

967. Take Your Minerals: One study linked a history of miscarriage to low levels of magnesium. Symptoms of magnesium deficiency can include agitation and anxiety, restless leg syndrome, sleep disorders, irritability, nausea, vomiting, abnormal heart rhythms, low blood pressure, confusion, muscle spasm and weakness, hyperventilation, insomnia, and even seizures. Foods high in magnesium include spinach, brown rice and pumpkin seeds.

968. Make Sure You Are Getting Enough Iron: Lack of iron has been reported to cause miscarriages. You may want to talk with your your doctor or nutritionist about taking an iron supplement. Food sources of iron include red meat, turkey, chicken, kidney beans and chick peas. Be sure you are taking Vitamin C to help iron absorption.

969. Take Baby Aspirin: Some studies have shown that taking one baby aspirin a day can reduce the risk of miscarriage. Ask your doctor about this. One of the benefits of baby aspirin is that it prevents blood clots that can cut off nutrients to the baby and prevents preeclampsia.

970. Be Alert To High Or Low Blood Pressure: Be sure you are aware of your blood pressure levels. Avoid fried or processed foods, deep breath and get plenty of rest. Repeat the word 'relax' several times a day.

971. Keep Blood Sugar Levels Stabile: Avoid sugar and do not let your blood sugar levels fluctuate. Your goal while pregnant is to maintain stable blood sugar levels. Avoid white flour, carbohydrates and sugar products that spike blood sugar levels.

972. Consider Taking Coenzyme Q10 Supplement: Research has shown that women with low levels of coenzyme q10 are at an increased risk of miscarriage.

973. Zinc: In some studies, zinc deficiency has been linked to miscarriage. Be sure your prenatal vitamin contains zinc. Symptoms of a zinc deficiency include frequent colds and infections, white spots on fingernails, mental exhaustion, poor appetite, dry skin and hair, poor sense of taste and smell. Natural sources of zinc include pumpkin seeds, lean meat, whole grains and oysters.

974. Folic Acid: Some studies have shown that women deficient in folic acid have up to three times the risk of miscarriage compared to women who have adequate levels of folic acid in their system. Folic acid reduces homocysteine levels. Be sure you are taking a high-quality folic acid supplement.

975. High-Quality Prenatal Vitamin: Be sure to take a high-quality prenatal vitamin with minerals such selenium. Selenium is a powerful antioxidant that can prevent chromosome breakage and DNA damage. Natural sources of selenium include brazil nuts and sunflower seeds.

976. Eat Lots of Grapes and Cherries: These foods contain the flavonoid quercertin, which keeps particles in the blood from sticking together and forming microscopic clumps, which can reduce or sometimes even block, blood flow from mother-to-baby.

977. Get Lots and Lots of Rest: This is no time to play superwoman. Nor it is the time to try to prove something. Be generous with the amount of rest and sleep you give yourself. Don't for a moment feel guilty that you are not running around doing what you used to do. Your developing fetus is the priority right now. You have nothing to prove. Listen to what your body needs and relax. Don't push yourself when you are tired. Yes, that invitation to go out sounds great and you don't want to be a spoil sport and say no—but you are feeling run-down. Guess what? This is the time to assert your right to say no—for your own good and your baby's good. This is not the time to try to prove something and if someone insinuates that a pregnant women shouldn't be babying themselves, ignore them and stay home. Be careful of late night social engagements, and trips where you might become exhausted from traveling or not sleeping well in a strange bed or new location. Before you book a cruise or a trip to Europe, you might want to consider the stress flying and being in a new place might have on your pregnancy.

If you feel that commuting to work or working at all is too much, talk to your ob/gyn about getting a note that you are in need of some bed rest.

You might also want to delay taking on big home projects, like moving, remodeling, or painting. Your new kitchen floor can wait until after the baby is born. This is not the time to do anything too emotionally or physically demanding.

Reduce the hours you work, ask to work from home, hire someone to clean your house and stop doing most of the chores. Guilt be gone—this is the time in your life to allow yourself rest so your baby can develop and grow. Ignore anyone who tries to make you feel guilty or goes on and on about how they did everything they normally did while they were pregnant. You deserve rest and you need to do whatever possible to get it.

978. Drink Lots of Water: It can help flush toxins from your body and away from your baby. Be sure to drink pure, filtered water.

979. Do You Have A Mineral Deficiency?: If you've had a miscarriage or recurrent miscarriage, you might want to have a mineral deficiency test. Be sure you are taking minerals in the form of a prenatal vitamin or a mineral supplement. Ask your doctor about this.

980. Talk To Your Doctor About Vitex: Agnus Castus, also known as Vitex, has been known to help women who have experienced a miscarriage because of a luteal phase defect. Vitex stimulates the function of the pituitary gland which controls and balances hormones. It also increases progesterone production.

981. Stay Away From Toxic Metals and Toxic Chemicals: Reduce radiation exposure, by reducing time spent on laptops, hair dryers, cell phones, iPads. Do not use hair dyes or deodorants. Avoid exposure to insect repellants, disinfectants, cleaning products, paints and anything with gaseous fumes. Do not use plastic utensils or Styrofoam cups at this time.

982. Avoid Heavy Lifting or Vacuuming: Avoid any type of exercise that strains your lower back or could impact your abdomen.

983. Exercise Lightly and In Moderation: Nothing strenuous or aerobic at this time. Avoid any excessive physical activity that could elevate body temperature and reduce blood flow to the fetus. Avoid activities like skiing, horseback riding, and surfing, that may cause you to lose your balance and lead to an abdominal area injury.

984. Less Sex Please: If possible, engage in gentle intercourse, and avoid putting too much pressure on your abdominal area. In Chinese medicine, it is often recommended that a couple abstain from sex during the entire nine months of pregnancy.

985. Avoid Vaccinations of Any Kind While Pregnant: There are some reports that flu shots have been linked to miscarriage. It is best to avoid vaccines while pregnant.

986. Herbs to Help Maintain Pregnancy: It is best to check with your doctor or a nutritionist before taking herbs.

987. Reduce Your Work Load: If possible, can you take a leave from work? Reduce your commute and work from home? If you feel you need to reduce your work hours, talk to your doctor about obtaining medical permission to go on bed rest. If you have miscarried in the past, or are concerned about a possible miscarriage, your ob/gyn may be able to help you obtain legitimate medical documentation for a leave from work or a request for a reduction in hours or a work-from-home situation.

988. Eat or Juice Garlic: Garlic can boost immunity, reduce inflammation in the body, reduce infections and cut the risk of pre-eclampsia. It reduces harmful bacteria, fungi and viruses, as well as improves blood circulation. Do not, however, take large or excessive amounts of garlic, as it can interact negativity with certain medications, lower blood sugar levels and reduce iodine absorption, which could lead to hypothyroidism.

989. Eat Foods High In Antioxidants: These include blueberries, cranberries, artichokes, Red Delicious and Granny Smith apples.

990. Be Careful What You Eat At Restaurants: If there is any chance you are pregnant, stop eating all meats, salads, fruits and vegetables at restaurants. You don't want to take a chance on foods that could be contaminated, dirty or undercooked. Consider either reducing or eliminating entirely tacos, hamburgers, hot dogs, or sausage subs also.

991. Sit in The Sunshine: Make sure you have adequate levels of Vitamin D. Women with low levels of Vitamin D are at a higher risk of developing preeclampsia.

992. Avoid Infections: Infections to be aware of and try to avoid include chicken pox, bacterial vaginosis, Chlamydia, fifth disease, toxoplasmosis, trichomoniasis, rubella, herpes, group B strep, and listeriosis. Wash your hands often with soap and warm water, especially after you have touched raw meat, eggs, unwashed vegetables, dirt or soil, or have been in contact with someone who is ill, gotten saliva on your hands, changed a diaper, played with children, or handled pets, including hamsters and guinea pigs. Do not share eating or drinking utensils. Avoid situations where you will be exposed to flus and other illnesses. Do not touch or change cat litter. Avoid contact with rodents or hire a professional to get them out of your house. Have someone clean your refrigerator, as juices from packages of hot dogs or deli meat can sometimes leak.

993. Foods To Avoid Or Be Very Careful Of While Pregnant

• No Chinese food

• No uncooked sausages, salami and only pepperoni if it has been heated until steaming hot.

• No prepared salads from a deli, especially if they contain eggs, chicken, ham or seafood.

• Avoid buffet or picnic food that has been sitting out in the heat.

• No stuffing inside a chicken, turkey or other bird.

• No unpasteurized fresh squeezed juice

• Avoid transfats.

• Do not drink the water if you have a water softener in your home.

• Be careful for toxoplasmosis, that is catchable from unwashed vegetables and cat feces.

• No blue cheese

• No raw cookie dough

• Even if you buy hot dogs that have been pre-cooked, you want to reheat until steaming hot, as they could contain listeria

• In Chinese medicine, it is believed that you should not eat pineapple or papaya in early pregnancy, as they can heat up the body and cause uterine contractions.

• No Raw Meat: Undercooked beef or poultry should be avoided completely when pregnant. Be very careful about this. I would recommend that while pregnant, do not eat any beef or poultry you did not cook yourself. Do not order meat at restaurants and if eating at the home of a friend or family member, be very sure they cook their meat well. Avoid rare meat or uncooked meat. Undercooked meat should be avoided because of the risk of contamination with coliform bacteria, toxoplasmosis, and salmonella. Even if you like your meat raw, cook all meats very, very well.

• No Deli Meat: Deli meats have been known to be contaminated with listeria, which can cause miscarriage. It may be best to entirely avoid deli meat while pregnant. Listeria has the ability to cross the placenta and infect the baby, leading to infection or blood poisoning, which may be life-threatening. If you feel it absolutely necessary to eat deli meats, reheat or microwave them until they are steaming hot. Do not eat deli meat rare.

• Avoid sushi.

• Avoid Smoked Seafood: Refrigerated, smoked seafood often labeled as lox, nova style, kippered, or jerky should be avoided because it could be contaminated with listeria.

• Avoid Fish Exposed to Industrial Pollutants: Fish that might contain high levels of mercury should be avoided. Mercury consumed during pregnancy has been linked to developmental delays and brain damage. Some of these fish can include: shark, swordfish, king mackerel, and tilefish. Tuna should be eaten in moderation. It is recommended not more than six ounces a week.

Do not eat fish from contaminated lakes and rivers that may be exposed to high levels of polychlorinated biphenyls, which is primarily fish that comes from local lakes and streams. So if someone you know is a fishermen and brings you something they caught, say no thank you. These fish can include: bluefish, striped bass, salmon, pike, trout, and walleye. Contact the local health department or Environmental Protection Agency to determine which fish are safe to eat in your area.

• Avoid Raw Shellfish: If you eat seafood, it should be cooked well. The majority of seafood-borne illnesses are caused by undercooked shellfish, which includes oysters, clams, and mussels. Cooking helps prevent some types of infection, but it does not prevent the algae-related infections that are associated with red tides. Raw shellfish pose a concern for everybody, and should be avoided altogether during pregnancy.

• Avoid Soft Cheeses: Imported soft cheeses may contain the bacteria listeria, which can cause miscarriage. Avoid soft cheeses such as:

-Brie

-Camembert

-Roquefort

-No feta cheese, which means avoiding Greek salads, spinach pie, and other foods made with feta.

-Gorgonzola and Mexican style cheeses that include queso blanco and queso fresco.

If you are eating at a restaurant or a friend's home, be sure to inquire as to what cheeses are in the food. It might be best to avoid Mexican restaurants at this time.

• Avoid Unpasteurized Milk: Unpasteurized milk may contain a bacteria called listeria. Make sure that any milk you drink is pasteurized.

• No Pate: Refrigerated pate or meat spreads should be avoided because they may contain the bacteria listeria.

• No Caffeine: Several studies have reported that caffeine can cause miscarriages. This is, of course, a personal choice, but it might be best to stop all coffee at this time. Many experts recommend avoiding coffee during the first trimester of a pregnancy to avoid miscarriage. You'll need to get your energy boost from natural sources, such as drinking green juices and eating lots of vegetables. If you need coffee for work or a long commute to work, you might want to consider taking time off or taking a leave from work if possible.

Your ob/gyn may be able to give you the documentation needed to obtain this. Overall, it is best to stop all coffee during your pregnant.

• No Alcohol: There is NO amount of alcohol that is known to be safe during pregnancy, and therefore alcohol should be avoided during pregnancy.

• Avoid Vegetables Or Salads At Restaurants: Make sure all vegetables you eat are washed very well to avoid potential exposure to toxoplasmosis. At this time, it might be best not to eat vegetables or salads from restaurants. If you are eating at the home of a friend or family member, be sure that all salads and vegetables have been washed thoroughly.

• Avoid Undercooked Eggs: Make sure any eggs you eat are well-cooked. The egg yolks and whites should be firm. Raw eggs or any foods that contain raw eggs should be avoided because of the potential exposure to salmonella. Foods containing eggs should be refrigerated. Be sure all utensils and pans that contained eggs are washed very, very well before you use them again. Consider putting them twice through the dishwasher to be safe.

If you eat well-cooked eggs, they should be eaten immediately after cooking—do not eat if they were left out for any length of time.

If you are baking at this time, remember that the eggs in a recipe are not yet cooked, so do not lick the spoon!

Do not eat foods made with raw or partially-cooked eggs, such as:

-Hollandaise sauce

-Caesar salad dressing

-Some frostings, both store bought and homemade

-Eggnog

-Homemade ice cream

-Custards

• Avoid fast foods and fast food restaurants

• No chicken or turkey that has been pre-stuffed, because the raw juice can mix with the stuffing.

• Avoid Unpasteurized Foods: This can include mozzarella cheese, cottage cheese or skim milk.

• Be Careful of Herbal Tea. Some herbal teas can induce labor and be dangerous for pregnant woman. It is best to consult with a physician or a very-experienced nutritionist on herbal teas.

• No Liver: Avoid or eat very little liver. It contains high levels of Vitamin A which have been known to cause birth defects.

• Do Not Eat Artificial Sweeteners While Pregnant.

• No Raw Sprouts: Avoid raw sprouts, as they have been linked to salmonella outbreaks.

• Avoid Prepared Meals that Include Deli Meat, Turkey, Beef, Hot Dogs, or Chicken from a Restaurant, Supermarket.

• Avoid ordering sandwiches at restaurants, supermarkets, delis or take-out while pregnant.

995. How to Maximize Your Chances For Conception The Days Before and After An IVF

Before:

• Consider additional acupuncture treatments close to the time you are doing an IVF. Ideally, increase the number of acupuncture treatments the week of the IVF to two to four. If you can, have one also done the day before the procedure. Perhaps if you go once a week, consider increasing your appointments to two to three times within the seven days before an IVF. Research has shown that acupuncture improves blood flow to the ovaries and uterus, relaxes uterine spasms, and relaxes the nervous system.

996. In the weeks prior to an IVF, make sure you are eating well. This is not the time to splurge on foods with lots of sugar, trans fats, msg, or white flour. Consider increasing the amount of vegetables you take in, such as spinach and garlic.

997. Green tea is linked to increased fertility. The polyphenols and hypoxanthine in green tea can increase the percentages of viable embroyos. Some studies suggest drinking treen tea can also help eggs become more fertile.

998. Increase the amounts of healthy fat you consume. In a recent study, women who ate avocados, a healthy monounsatured fat, were more likely to conceive a child after IVF. Other healthy fats include olive oil. Avoid saturated fats and trans fats as much as you can, ideally entirely, for two to four weeks before IVF.

999. Be aware of the help certain supplements can provide, such as coenzyme Q10, which in some studies have shown to improve egg quality. Some studies have shown that women taking coenzyme Q10 had higher fertilization rates in IVF than women who weren't taking the supplement. Some studies also show that coenzyme Q10 deficiency can sometimes cause miscarriage.

1000. Increase your time spent in the sunshine to 30 minutes a day if you possibly can. Even if it is cold out, try to be in the sun more than usual amount of time. Perhaps bundle up and sit outside. Sunlight increases levels of Vitamin D, which is key to balancing sex hormones in women and improving sperm count in men, according to various researchers. In cold northern countries, the rate of conception increases during the summer months, according to some studies. If you are doing an IVF in the summer and you live near a beach, park or lake, consider spending more than the usual time outside in the sun.

1001. Pineapple contains a proteolytic enzyme called bromelain which reduces inflammation, improves uterine lining and breaks up proteins that prevent embryo implantation. Eating pineapple core a few days before an IVF cycle can help implantation. Cut the core into round sections and eat after embryo transfers to help implantation. Note: Stop eating pineapple after any IVF or IUI or if you think if there is any chance you might be pregnant. While pineapple helps implantation, it is not recommended for pregnancy.

1002. Close to the time of transfer, cut out all sugar and white flour products if you possibly can.

1003. Make sure your guy is eating garlic, raw pumpkin and sunflower seeds, walnuts, almonds, and oysters. Reduce his amount of dairy and fat.

1004. Stop all coffee and caffeine products close to the time of conception. Ideally, perhaps a week or two before an IVF.

1005. Make sure you are taking a prenatal vitamin and folic acid.

1006. About two weeks before the IVF, stop the late bedtimes and give yourself added sleep.

1007. Do whatever you can to start to relax. Spend more time in nature, knit, crochet, listen to soothing music, get a massage. Take a break from thinking about all your problems. As much as you can, get your body out of fight or flight mode.

1008. If it is summer and you live near a beach, consider a week-long beach vacation a week before your IVF and a week after the IVF. The time spent relaxing, in the sunshine, might help your body prepare for pregnancy.

After the IUI/IVF:

1009. For a few days, make sure you get adequate sleep and try to keep stress levels down. Whatever you can do to promote a deep feeling of relaxation, do it. If that means, spending a day just sitting by the ocean, singing, or doing some art work that relaxes you. The goal is to let yourself feel peace. I know this is easier said than done, especially when so much is riding on the outcome of an IVF. And to be frank, many women get pregnant stressed or not, so don't get into a doomsday mode if you simply can't relax. The human body is strong and can often conceive even in bad circumstances. But whatever you can do to relax and reduce stress levels, be open to doing. Knit, crochet, watch something funny that makes you laugh. Spend time in nature, whether at the beach, a lake, a beautiful park, your backyard or just sitting outside in a driveway.

1010. Make sure you continue to get adequate amounts of sunshine each day.

1011. If you can plan a getaway, not too far from your home, during the wait time after an IVF, that might help. A getaway to a local beach, lake, something relaxing that doesn't take a lot of planning or travel time. Do not go away if travel in any way makes you feel stressed or overwhelmed. Something within an hour's drive might be ideal.

1012. If you can, take a few days or even a week off of work to just be home, rest, listen to music, and have fun.

1013. Continue to eat foods that promote fertility. Olive oil, avocado, spinach.

1014. Stay away from screens as much as you can.

1015. Ask your doctor about progesterone and if you might need it to help implantation.

1016. Don't drink coffee.

1017. Avoid hot baths.

1018. Keep positive and see yourself as pregnant. Try to keep a hopeful, happy outlook.

Repeat affirmations like:
I welcome you baby.
Life is beautiful.
I am pregnant.
My body is comfortable receiving.
It is safe for me to be pregnant.
 It is safe for me to have a baby.
I give myself permission to be pregnant.
I am allowed to get pregnant.
I am ready to be pregnant.

Write, say and sing these words as often as you can.